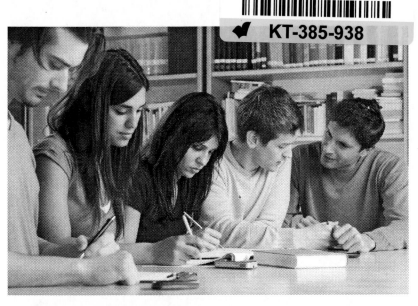

Succeeding in your Medical School Application

How to prepare the perfect UCAS Personal Statement

Third Edition

Matt Green

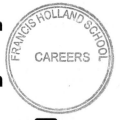

BPP

Francis Holland School NW1 6XR

First edition 2007
Third edition March 2012

ISBN 9781 4453 8166 4
Previous ISBN 9781 9068 3905 5
e-ISBN 9781 4453 9389 6

British Library Cataloguing-in-Publication Data
A catalogue record for this book is available from
the British Library

Published by
BPP Learning Media Ltd
BPP House, Aldine Place
London W12 8AA

www.bpp.com/health

Typeset by Replika Press Pvt Ltd, India
Printed in the United Kingdom

Your learning materials, published by BPP
Learning Media Ltd, are printed on paper
sourced from sustainable, managed forests.

The views expressed in this book are those of
BPP Learning Media and not those of UCAS or
any medical school. BPP Learning Media are in
no way associated with or endorsed by UCAS or
any medical school.

The contents of this book are intended as a guide
and not professional advice. Although every effort
has been made to ensure that the contents of
this book are correct at the time of going to
press, BPP Learning Media, the Editor and the
Author make no warranty that the information
in this book is accurate or complete and accept
no liability for any loss or damage suffered by
any person acting or refraining from acting as a
result of the material in this book.

Every effort has been made to contact the
copyright holders of any material reproduced
within this publication. If any have been
inadvertently overlooked, BPP Learning Media
will be pleased to make the appropriate credits
in any subsequent reprints or editions.

ii

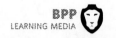

Contents

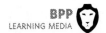

Contents

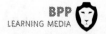

About the Publisher

BPP Learning Media is dedicated to supporting aspiring professionals with top quality learning material. BPP Learning Media's commitment to success is shown by our record of quality, innovation and market leadership in paper-based and e-learning materials. BPP Learning Media's study materials are written by professionally-qualified specialists who know from personal experience the importance of top quality materials for success.

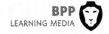

Reaching your Goal

The process of applying to medical school can be a somewhat long and arduous process but the rewards of a career within Medicine are infinite. BPP Learning Media and BPP University College School of Health are committed to supporting aspiring and current doctors to progress their career through our comprehensive range of books, personal development courses and degree programmes. I often say there is no other vocation that provides such breadth and depth of career options for the individual to follow and specialise in. Whether it is the fast paced nature of the A&E department or the measured environment of Pathology, there is something for everyone.

There is no greater privilege than being responsible for leading the treatment of patients and sharing in their recovery. There are few other careers that provide such diversity on a daily basis. A passion for helping others, clear communication skills especially empathy, excellent team working and leadership qualities as well as the ability to strike a work-life balance are all skills that an accomplished doctor should possess.

The decision to follow a career in Medicine is something that should not be taken lightly and you should undertake careful research to ensure it really is for you. A career in Medicine is not for everyone and I would urge readers to ensure they have undertaken sufficient work experience to gain a balanced insight into what becoming a doctor really entails.

I first began mentoring aspiring medical students seven years ago when it was clear that many individuals were not gaining access to the help and support they required to successfully apply to medical school. It was with this in mind that I embarked on publishing our Entry to Medical School Series to provide a clear insight into the various facets of successfully getting into medical school. Whether it is help with choosing the

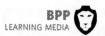

right medical school, how to prepare an outstanding personal statement or how to succeed in your medical school interview, our comprehensive range of books provide the advice that is so often hard to find.

I would like to take this opportunity to wish you the very best of luck with applying to medical school and hope that you pass on some of the gems of wisdom that you acquire along the way to other aspiring medics.

Matt Green
Series Editor – Entry to Medical School
Medical Publishing Director

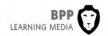

About the Author

Matt Green BSc (Hons) MPhil

Matt Green has spent the last six years directly helping over 5,000 individuals successfully apply to medical school. It is with this extensive experience in mind that Matt has written this book to help prospective medical students prepare their UCAS personal statement as part of their application to medical school.

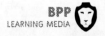

Acknowledgements

I would like to thank all the students who have helped to make this book a reality together with a special thanks to Nicola for her ongoing support.

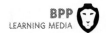

Preface

'What makes a good doctor?

Clearly someone who communicates well, empathises with patients and exercises sound clinical judgement. But a doctor should also understand the basic mechanisms of disease, be able to test hypotheses and show curiosity and a capacity for self-directed learning. Teaching reinforces these scientific principles and an Oxford doctor is trained to be a good scientist as well as a good clinician and a clear thinker.'

(Oxford University website, June 2007)

This informative guide is intended to help applicants to medical schools in the United Kingdom submit an effective, compelling Personal Statement. It will assist school leavers, graduates and mature applicants alike, as well as parents and teachers. Please use this guide alongside advice provided by your school or college, from the Universities and College Admissions Service, and assistance offered by the medical schools themselves.

This guide includes examples from real and fictitious 'Personal Statements' in order to illustrate certain key principles. It is vitally important that you see them as they are – illustrative examples.

The most important aspect of your Personal Statement is that it is written by, and is about, you!

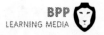

Chapter 1

Applying to a medical school in the United Kingdom: The process

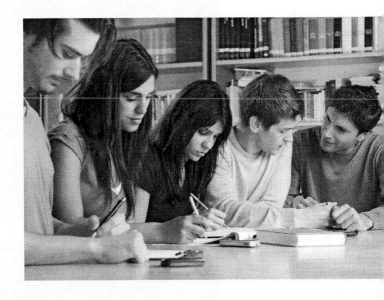

Applying to a medical school in the United Kingdom: The process

In 2012 there were 93,581 applications to study Medicine and Dentistry in the United Kingdom (source: www.ucas.com/about_us/media_enquiries/media_releases/2011/20111128). Across the country, there are on average around five applications for each medical school place on offer.

There are three steps in this application process:

- Sitting the appropriate entrance examination where applicable. (Examinations take place between June and October in the year before successful candidates begin their medical studies).

- Submitting a university application which includes the Personal Statement (mid-October deadline).

- Attending a selection interview when applicable. (Interviews take place between October and the following June depending upon the medical school).

Medical school entrance examinations

An increasing number of medical schools require candidates to complete an entrance examination before submitting their actual application. It is therefore important to determine as soon as possible whether or not the medical schools to which you intend to apply require you to sit an entrance examination. Those in current use are based upon an aptitude format assessing a number of different criteria. The aim of these tests is to aid the application process by ensuring that appropriate attitude, mental competence and professional qualities are specifically considered.

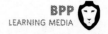

Presently there are three examination formats in use in the UK:

- United Kingdom Clinical Aptitude Test (UKCAT)
- Biomedical Admissions Test (BMAT)
- Graduate Medical Schools Admissions Test (GAMSAT)

The closing dates for these tests differ and we advise you to consult the relevant websites listed in the following sections for more information.

UKCAT

The UKCAT aptitude test was formally adopted in 2006 by 23 of the medical schools in the UK. The test is designed to assist admissions tutors select candidates who possess the desired mental abilities, approaches and attributes of successful medical students and practising doctors.

The test sets out to examine the following five qualities:

- Verbal reasoning
- Quantitative reasoning
- Abstract reasoning
- Decision analysis
- Non-cognitive analysis

For more information visit: **www.ukcat.ac.uk**

BMAT

The BMAT aptitude test is currently used by a number of medical schools, including Cambridge, Oxford, Imperial College and University College, London.

The test covers three sections:

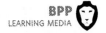

- Section 1   This evaluates generic skills which are important for effective undergraduate study. These include complex problem-solving techniques, evaluating balanced arguments, and the ability to analyse data.

- Section 2   This is restricted to topics in mathematics and science.

- Section 3   This normally comprises a short essay.

For more information and advice regarding the BMAT test visit: **www.bmat.org.uk**

GAMSAT

The GAMSAT aptitude test was developed by the Australian Council for Medical Research and is specifically used in the consideration of graduate applicants to medical schools. Among the UK universities which use the GAMSAT test are the University of Wales and Nottingham University.

The GAMSAT test evaluates:

- Practical experience, attributes and skills
- Knowledge and implementation of concepts in basic science
- Problem-solving, critical thinking and writing skills

For more information and advice regarding the GAMSAT test visit: **www.gamsat-ie.org/**

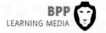

The UCAS application

As the competition for medical school places continues to increase, the need for a clear, engaging and well-structured university application is paramount. The Universities and Colleges Admission Service (UCAS) mediate applications made to universities in the United Kingdom through an online system (for more information visit www.ucas.com). If you are at school or college, the application process will be co-ordinated by the head of post-16 education and you will be provided with login details and instructions on how to proceed. If you are applying as a graduate or mature student not currently in full time education, you can register with UCAS directly in order to submit your application.

You cannot apply directly to a UK medical school to study Medicine. All applications must be made via UCAS using the somewhat daunting 'UCAS application form' which is now in electronic format. Although the paper-based 'UCAS form' is not commonly used now for applications to medical school, the electronic application process still requires all of the information that would have been previously submitted. Accordingly, the electronic UCAS form requires you to enter your personal details, your course choices, your predicted or actual grades, your reference and your Personal Statement.

When considering an application to medical school, the admissions tutors place particular emphasis upon your entrance examination result (where applicable), academic performance, your reference and your Personal Statement. Indeed, some medical schools currently make offers to students based solely on their applications without conducting any interviews.

At present, the medical school Personal Statement must be completed within 4,000 characters. It is also important to note that when entering the Personal Statement onto the UCAS system, any formatting – such as underlining, italics or bolding – will be lost.

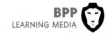

So, your UCAS Personal Statement is your key opportunity to convince medical school admissions tutors that you are an exceptional candidate and that they should offer you a place at their medical school over other applicants.

It is vital that you make your comments clearly and compellingly, so that the admissions tutors become really keen to meet you and find out more about this special, unique person that you are!

Applying to study different subjects

Currently, candidates applying to study Medicine are restricted to applying to four medical schools in a calendar year whereas applicants for degree subjects other than Medicine are invited to apply to six universities. Accordingly, applicants to study Medicine are also able to apply for two other non-medical courses, such as Pharmacy or Biomedical Sciences. However it is important to remember that within each candidate's application, only one Personal Statement can be submitted.

It is the advice of the authors, based upon their practical experience, that candidates seeking to study Medicine should write their Personal Statement wholly with the aim of gaining acceptance to study Medicine. Any attempt to incorporate other course choices would be inadvisable; such an approach would almost certainly reduce the strength of the Personal Statement.

KEY POINTS
- Make sure that you first make contact with UCAS, the entrance examinations websites, and the medical schools themselves in order to find out exactly what you need to do when applying to study Medicine.

- Attending university Open Days is especially valuable; you have the chance then to ask questions directly.

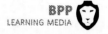

Chapter 2

What kind of students do medical schools want?

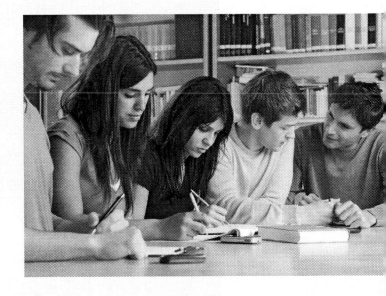

What kind of students do medical schools want?

The Council of Heads of Medical Schools, in consultation with the Department of Health and British Medical Association, have produced a statement setting out guiding principles for the selection and admission of students to medical schools.

These are:

1. **Selection for medical school implies selection for the medical profession**

   A degree in Medicine confirms academic achievement and in normal circumstances entitles the new graduate to be provisionally registered by the General Medical Council.

2. The selection process attempts to identify the core academic and non-academic qualities of a doctor:

   • **Honesty, integrity** and an ability to **recognise one's own limitations** and those of others, are central to the practice of medicine.

   • Other key attributes include having **good communication** and **listening skills**, an ability **to make decisions under pressure**, and to **remain calm and cope with stress**.

   • Doctors must have an understanding of **teamwork** and respect for the contributions of others. Desirable characteristics include **curiosity, creativity, initiative, flexibility** and **leadership**.

3. A high level of academic attainment will be expected. **Understanding science is core to the understanding of medicine**, but medical schools generally encourage diversity in subjects studied by candidates.

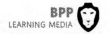

4.   The practice of medicine requires the highest standards of **professional** and **personal conduct**. Put simply, some students will not be suited to a career in medicine and it is in the interests of the student and the public that they should not be admitted to medical school.

5.   The practice of medicine requires the highest standards of **professional competence**. However, a history of serious ill health or disability will not jeopardise a career in medicine unless the condition impinges upon professional fitness to practise.

6.   Candidates should demonstrate some understanding of what a career in medicine involves and their suitability for a caring profession.

Medical schools expect candidates to have had some relevant experience in health or related areas. Indeed, some medical schools stipulate a defined minimum period of relevant work experience.

7.   The **primary duty of care is to patients**. All applicants to medical schools will be expected to understand the importance of this principle.

8.   Failure to declare information that has a material influence on a student's fitness to practise may lead to termination of their medical course.

Clearly, it is important that you consult the websites of the medical schools to which you intend to apply in order to learn of any specific requirements they are seeking.

University education is also expensive. For every medical student who drops out, there are financial implications to the university. **So, one of the most important questions to be considered by a medical school is: will the student complete the course?**

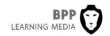

Finally, medical schools are also looking for students who will contribute to the broad spectrum of university life. Those who do so are so much more likely to gain a wider experience of working and communicating with people from different backgrounds.

The admissions tutor's perspective

In deciding who will and who will not to be invited to study Medicine at their university, medical schools look to the views of their admissions tutors, the people who read the application submissions and who conduct the interviews.

And when reading hundreds of Personal Statements, so often the key considerations of the tutors are:

> *'Does this candidate have a sense of what they are going to get into by studying Medicine, and indeed by studying Medicine at this medical school?'*

> *'Can I see this individual becoming a good practising doctor in a few years from now?'*

While it is likely that admissions tutors will be looking to see if you possess the personal qualities so often associated with doctors – qualities such as kindness, compassion, empathy, and curiosity – they are perhaps even more determined to see if you are always reliable, and that you can handle the physical, mental and emotional strains you will experience, firstly as a medical student and then as a professional practitioner.

KEY POINTS
- Selection for medical school implies selection for the medical profession.
- Medical schools want candidates with more than academic ability. They want to train the doctors of tomorrow.

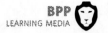

Chapter 3

The essential contents of the Personal Statement

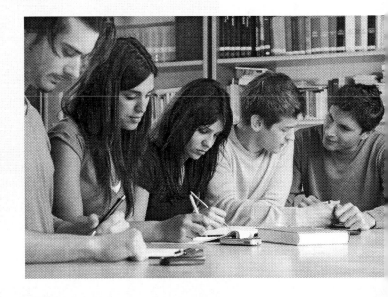

Chapter 3

The essential contents of the Personal Statement

Your Personal Statement is your opportunity to describe in words:

- The reasons why you are so keen to study Medicine, and at the universities to which you are submitting your applications.

- That even in advance of taking up your medical studies, you have already made a real commitment to this course of action by gaining relevant experience.

- That you have a good idea of, and are equipped to handle, the expectations, responsibilities, pressures and duties attached to the practice of medicine.

- That you are special, and possess attributes which will see you through your medical course and towards establishing your medical professional career.

Let us take each of these themes above and look at them carefully.

What is Medicine?

Medicine offers a broad range of careers from general practice to the specialties of hospital practice and to medical research. Medicine is an applied science, but it is equally about dealing sympathetically and effectively with individuals, whether they be patients or colleagues. Medicine increasingly poses difficult ethical dilemmas, and, above all, medicine is constantly and rapidly developing and providing a stimulating challenge to practitioners and medical scientists alike.

(Oxford University website, June 2007)

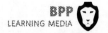

Every would-be medical student has their own story as to how and why they came to make that academic and career choice. In your Personal Statement, it is vital that you explain **your** own journey in **your** own **unique** way. But you must present your story with real **conviction**.

In 2006, editors of the British Medical Journal asked three doctors who are responsible for some of the most inspiring medical textbooks to write upon the theme of 'Why medicine inspires me?' (BMJ Vol 333, 23-30th Dec 2006, pgs 1320-1323. The following extracts are reproduced with permission from the BMJ Publishing Group.) Their accounts are incredibly illuminating and written with great passion.

Here are some of their comments:

> *'As is hopefully true for all doctors, I am inspired by the opportunity to spend my professional lifetime trying to improve the health and welfare of humanity. I always believed that no higher calling existed than to help individual patients.'*

> *'I find it hard to look back and capture what initially inspired me to take up medicine, but I think that my aspirations are still the same. Medicine is a "way of life" and combines that rather nebulous feeling of wanting to help and care with the more exact principles of science and logical thought. After all these years as a doctor, I still want to get out of bed and go to work in the mornings.'*

> *'Doctors are at the top of the list of professions that the public thinks are worthy of "respect" and also are "most likely to tell the truth", and this makes me feel privileged to be a doctor.'*

> *'There is no place for arrogance or self-satisfaction. I still relish a diagnostic conundrum that calls on all my faculties and training to tease it out. I have been fortunate to treat people from different ethnic groups with different cultures, beliefs and*

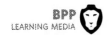

diseases. This has been a humbling experience but also educational and fascinating.'

'Medicine offers a huge variety of choices – clinical work, research, teaching, training and management – to name but a few. Medicine is currently undergoing many changes. The medical curriculum has changed almost beyond recognition since I was a student. More emphasis is placed on communication and clinical skills. The greatest joy is that simple "thank you" as the patient walks out of the door. Isn't it great?'

'Medicine is based on altruism, science, and human interest. Like most medical students, this is what attracted me and it still does. The aspirations are of excellent care, progress, and change. I find the continuing movement, and certainty that we will know more, inspirational and energising. Medicine is remarkable in its clinical and scientific breadth and its fusion with other disciplines and interests. Much of medicine grows from basic biology, but medical research and practice is also linked to physics, chemistry, statistics, population science, sociology and politics. It is remarkable, for example, that new technical platforms allow quick identification of genetic patterns that in future may influence treatment given to individual patients and that this, in turn, will raise ethical and political issues for society at large.'

'Whatever interests and personality you have, there is probably an aspect of medicine to suit you. The diversity can be confusing for a student and young doctor thinking about a career. When I qualified I did not know what would be the best path to choose.'

'Teaching and training are essential components of medicine. Brilliant lectures and articles and new discoveries and ideas are great rejuvenators. Cancer medicine has been a constant source of inspiration. Few areas of medicine demand the same degree of technical expertise and human understanding. The constant development of new approaches is engrossing.'

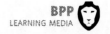

Clearly, these accounts are written with the wisdom which comes after many years of medical experience. But the statements really do deserve careful consideration; they were written by doctors, to be read, very largely, by other doctors.

For example, look at the ways these authors describe their enthusiasm for medicine: in particular, note the use of words such as *'inspired'*, *'aspirations'*, *'relish'*, *'energising'*, *'engrossing'*.

Look also at their references to the challenges and uncertainties which accompany medical studies. For example,

'The diversity can be confusing for a student' and *'When I qualified I did not know what would be the best path to choose'*.

When writing your own Personal Statement, you must write in your own style. However, you can be sure that admissions tutors are looking to see evidence of **enthusiasm** and careful **reflection** in your comments.

Why Medicine at this university?

Before you begin to write your medical school Personal Statement you need to decide the medical schools to which you wish to apply. It is important that you consult a careers advisor and visit the medical schools yourself before making your final decision. This is a decision not to be taken lightly given the fact that you will be dedicating the next several years to studying there.

There are many factors to take into account when considering your choice, including:

• Would you prefer to study at a campus or city-based medical school?

• Do you feel comfortable in the locality in which the medical school is set?

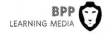

- Are you happy with the educational approaches taken by the medical schools under consideration? These do vary. For example, some courses concentrate on problem-based learning, a style of teaching which is based on the consideration of case studies, or scenarios, and the students presenting their findings in the context of achieving defined educational objectives.

- When would you start interacting with patients?

- What extra-curricular activities are available?

- Do you want to study close to your family home, or not?

Each medical school has a slightly different selection process so it is important that you also visit their website in order to obtain the necessary details.

Your commitment to medical studies and a medical career

Consider the situation in which a Premier League football club is deliberating whether or not to offer a teenage boy, with aspirations to be a professional footballer, a position within the club's youth academy. You can be sure that in addition to their consideration of his football ability, the club's coaches will also be looking to see signs of a real commitment to a future career in the sport as demonstrated by, for example, his approach to diet, and his attitude to drinking and smoking. In short, the club will be keen to see evidence of personal investment in this career move. What is he keen to do; what is he prepared to give up?

The same applies in the consideration of medical school applications. The admissions tutors will be keen to find out how you spend your time outside the formal school curriculum.

For example, they may look to see if your Personal Statement contains evidence that:

- You try to keep abreast of medical developments as they are reported in leading medical journals (for example, *The Lancet*, the *BMJ*) and the national newspapers, or

- You spend time at weekends supporting staff in a local hospice, care home or hospital.

Understanding the expectations, responsibilities and duties attached to the practice of medicine

The most authoritative description of the responsibilities and duties of doctors working in the United Kingdom is that issued by the General Medical Council (GMC), the body with which all medical practitioners in our country must become registered.

Presented below is the statement from the GMC defining the duties of a doctor taken from 'Good Medical Practice'. **It is imperative that all applicants to medical school gain a full understanding of the GMC's requirements.**

The duties of a doctor registered with the General Medical Council

Patients must be able to trust doctors with their lives and health. To justify that trust you must show respect for human life. And you must:

- *Make the care of patients your first concern*
- *Protect and promote the health of patients and the public*
- *Provide a good standard of practice and care*
  - *Keep your professional knowledge and skills up to date*
  - *Recognise and work within the limits of your professional competence*
  - *Work with colleagues in the ways that best serve patients' interests*

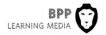

- *Treat patients as individuals and respect their dignity*
    - *Treat patients politely and considerately*
    - *Respect patients' right to confidentiality*

- *Work in partnership with patients*
    - *Listen to patients and respond to their concerns and preferences*
    - *Give patients the information they want and in a way they can understand*
    - *Respect patients' right to reach decisions with you about their treatment and care*
    - *Support patients in caring for themselves to improve and maintain their health*

- *Be honest and trustworthy*
    - *Act without delay if you have good reason to believe that you or a colleague may be putting patients at risk*
    - *Never discriminate unfairly against patients or colleagues*
    - *Never abuse your patients' trust in you or the public's trust in the profession*

You are personally accountable for your professional practice and must always be prepared to justify your decisions and actions.

Accordingly, by drawing upon your experiences in life, especially your work experience, it is vital that you use your Personal Statement to convince the admissions tutors that you are able to:

- Engage appropriately with ill or disabled people, and
- Listen to them and to support them, and
- Work effectively as a member of a team.

Remember, *'there is no place for arrogance or self-satisfaction'* and that setting a course upon becoming a doctor is a *'humbling experience'*.

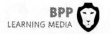

It is also important that you indicate your understanding of the physical and emotional demands placed upon medical students and doctors. It is indeed a *'way of life'*: doctors are so often seen as role models for society.

Finally, by all means indicate where your specific medical career interests might presently lie but also understand that your views may well change in the light of your medical education and clinical experiences.

Show them you are special

When considering the Personal Statements of applicants to medical schools, the admissions tutors will also be asking themselves:

- *Has this applicant really thought things through?*
- *Do we want to meet this candidate at interview?*
- *Do we see them enjoying and completing their studies, well on their way to becoming a good doctor?*
- *Will it be good for the university to have this candidate around?*

Your Personal Statement is your opportunity to influence the tutors towards saying 'Yes' in response to each of these questions as they apply to you!

So, it is important that you write in a way that depicts the enthusiasm, keenness – and indeed, **passion** – you have for your chosen academic choice.

Phrases such as 'I am *quite* interested in studying Medicine' or 'I really *think* that Medicine is the right course for me' are to be avoided; they are so unconvincing! And if you have received special commendations or prizes, write about them in a way that shows how they reinforce your decision to study Medicine.

For example, if you became Head Pupil at your school, this clearly shows the strength of the teachers' regard for your leadership

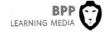

qualities, and your ability to act as a role model for other pupils. So, elaborate upon those themes. Equally, if you worked effectively as part of a team raising money for your school's charity you could describe how this experience improved your teamwork and communication skills.

It is vitally important when referring to your experiences in your Personal Statement to clearly state how these have developed in you the qualities that are required of a medical student and future doctor.

However, before you submit your final statement, you would also do well to talk about your 'special' qualities with your referee. Some comments are simply more effectively made by another person and it is important that your reference fully supports your application to medical school.

KEY POINT
It is vital that you use your medical school Personal Statement to convince the admissions tutors that you have really considered the implications of studying Medicine and that you know it is right for you.

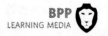

Chapter 4

Medical school applications: The myths

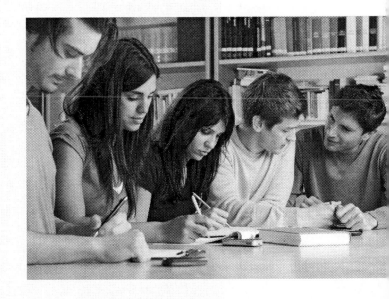

Medical school applications: The myths

During my experience in supporting students in their applications to medical schools, I have come across many misunderstandings. Here are some which arise time after time:

1. **Medical schools are keen to meet students whose key motivation for wishing to become a doctor is due to a parent being a doctor.**

    No. Clearly, the fact that one of your parents is a doctor may very significantly account for your keen interest in studying Medicine. However, this is simply not sufficient justification for your decision to embark upon a medical career. Admissions tutors will be looking to see how you have carefully considered your career options, and how you have confirmed your final choice by gaining appropriate experience.

2. **It is easier to get into medical school if your parent is a doctor.**

    This is not true. Again, if your parent is a doctor it is certainly easier to gain an insight into the world of medicine. However, medical schools are interested in each individual applicant and in the steps they have undertaken to confirm that they have the right qualities for a future medical career.

3. **Medical schools are much more likely to take students from private schools.**

    This is simply not true – medical schools look to offer places to the best candidates regardless of whether they attended a private or state school. Your suitability for gaining an interview and subsequent place will be determined by the quality of your university application, including particularly the effort that you have placed in preparing your Personal Statement. Remember, together with your predicted grades,

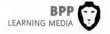

it is predominantly the strength of your Personal Statement and your reference that will determine whether you are invited to attend an interview or not.

4. **I am the first person to ever apply to medical school from my school, therefore I don't stand a chance of getting in.**

    This is not true and a common misconception. Simply because you may be the first person from your school or college to apply to study Medicine does not mean that your chances are reduced. Successful candidates are those who have invested time and effort in preparing their applications, and who have ensured that their referees became aware of their keen intentions to study Medicine.

5. **I must achieve all A grades in my GCSEs and my A levels to get into medical school.**

    This is not necessarily true and depends on the particular medical school and its entry requirements. It is therefore important that you carefully study the admissions criteria of the medical schools to which you intend to apply.

6. **Despite my greatest efforts I have been unable to secure work experience in a medical setting therefore I will not be able to apply to medical school.**

    Although for some people it may be difficult to secure work experience within a hospital or general practice surgery, there are many other options open to you that will enable you to gain first-hand experience of working with ill or disabled people. These include working:

    *   At a care or nursing home
    *   In a hospice
    *   Within a voluntary organisation, such as St John Ambulance or Samaritans

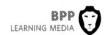

- With support groups for the disabled

Remember, your work experience is crucial in enabling you to obtain first-hand experience of working with, and helping to improve the quality of life of, ill or disabled people, and confirming that you have what it takes to follow this through and establish a medical career.

7. **Scoring well in my examinations is the only thing I need to do to get into medical school.**

Not true at all. Yes, successful applicants to medical schools will obtain excellent academic results; however, it is vital that they also demonstrate that they have the qualities required of a good doctor. Think back to your own experiences when you were treated by a doctor: what special qualities made them stand out? Some of these include:

- Having a real desire to help people
- Being able to communicate clearly
- Understanding the importance of effective team working and leadership skills
- Being empathic and honest
- Recognising the importance of adopting a conscientious and highly motivated approach

8. **When describing your work experience you should not refer to non-medical experience.**

It is important to refer to your medical and your non-medical experiences to demonstrate how these have helped to equip you in your forthcoming studies, and beyond. For example, someone describing that they had led a mountaineering expedition would clearly demonstrate their strong leadership and team working skills.

9. **My Personal Statement must be exactly 4,000 characters or I will be penalised.**

    Obviously, the more relevant information you include within the allowed space then the more fully you will be able to tell the admissions tutors about yourself and why you should be offered a place at their medical school. However, it really is about quality not quantity, so do not attempt to pad out your Personal Statement with irrelevant facts that do not add any value to your application or, worse still, weaken it.

10. **The sooner I submit my Personal Statement before the deadline the better my chances of success.**

    This is another common misconception. The only real advantage of submitting your medical school application as early as possible is that it will reduce your stress levels and enable you to concentrate on your studies. Despite what is commonly perceived, submitting your application earlier rather than later will not mean that you stand a better chance of your application progressing simply because it is at the top of the admission tutor's pile!

11. **If I select one other course choice in addition to Medicine I will reduce my chances.**

    Admissions tutors will not think that you are less committed to studying Medicine if you list one other course in addition to the four medical school applications you have submitted. Indeed, unless the courses you have selected are at the same university, the Data Protection Act precludes admissions tutors the ability to identify your other applications.

However, it is important that your Personal Statement is 100% tailored to your application to study Medicine and does not contain reference to other non-medical courses.

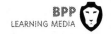

KEY POINT

Your Personal Statement is your opportunity to justify to the admissions tutors why you, as a unique individual, should be accepted to medical school in the first step of a medical career.

Chapter 5

Preparing your Personal Statement

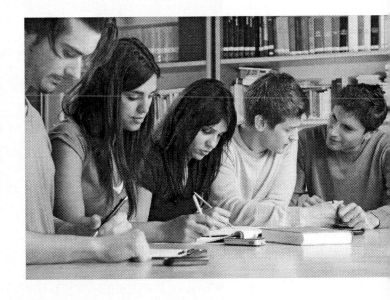

Preparing your Personal Statement

Check the key questions

The first step in preparing your Personal Statement is to take a good look at yourself – your personality, your strengths and your achievements. Then take a blank piece of paper and write down where you stand with regard to the key questions set out below. It is almost certain that you will not be able to touch upon each and every topic covered by these questions in your final Personal Statement. However, it will be helpful for you to consider each question; you can then decide which areas you are keen to include and which ones you are content to discard.

You might also find it valuable to have to hand the following when considering the key questions below:

- The list of 'Duties of a doctor registered with the General Medical Council' (page 17)

- The guiding principles for the admission of medical students formulated by the Council of Heads of Medical Schools (page 8) and

- The quotations relating to 'Why medicine inspires me' (page 13)

But please note: it is extremely important that when it comes to writing your Personal Statement, you create your own expressions and phrases. Your Personal Statement has to be written uniquely in your style – about you!

Key questions
- When and why did you begin to be interested in Medicine?

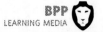

- Why do you want to study Medicine? Are you sure you want to be a doctor? Why do you want to be a doctor rather than, for example, a nurse, or a physiotherapist? Or a lawyer?

- Why are you so keen to study Medicine at this particular university?

- What kind of person are you? Which aspects of your personality equip you well for medical studies and a career in medicine?

- What are your strengths and weaknesses? What are your strengths and weaknesses according to others, such as your parents, your friends, your teachers? What special talents do you have which could be of real value within a medical career?

- What work experience have you had which has given you a special insight into life as a medical student or as a doctor?

- What else have you done, or has happened to you, which has provided excellent learning experiences or drawn upon your special personal qualities, such as compassion, tenacity, empathy?

- What awards or prizes (academic and non-academic) have you received? What do these tell people about you?

- What are your keen interests outside academic studies?

- What do you see yourself doing in five or ten years' time.

Drafting a structure

When complete, an effective Personal Statement will comprise three key sections: your 'introduction', a 'conclusion', and

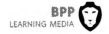

between these two sections will lie those paragraphs comprising the 'main body' of the Personal Statement.

It is helpful to sketch onto a piece of blank paper three boxes; one labelled 'Introduction', one labelled 'Conclusion' and, lying between those two boxes, one labelled 'Main body'.

Now start mapping some draft comments to each of the three sections.

The introduction

The aim of the introduction is to catch the attention of the reader, namely the admissions tutor. So, try to compose a statement which really grabs the reader's attention and enables you to stand out from the crowd!

The main body of the Personal Statement

The main body of your Personal Statement is the section in which you build upon your introduction and describe:

- Why you have decided to study Medicine

- The steps you have taken in making a real commitment to study Medicine

- How you have a real sense of what medical studies and a subsequent medical career entail

- Aspects of yourself which especially equip you for this course of action

It is in this section that you will refer to:

- Your work experience, and the relevant insights it has given you towards confirming that studying Medicine is right for you

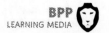

- The steps you have taken in furthering your interest in Medicine and medical matters

- The topics which you look forward to studying most

- Your experience of teamwork, leadership and responsibility, reliability and tenacity

- Your thoughts upon what direction your medical career might take, always recognising that this might change in the light of experience at medical school.

The conclusion

It is vitally important to draw your Personal Statement to a close, and reaffirm that you are someone who will flourish academically and socially at medical school, and that you are well equipped to handle the stresses and strains associated with medical studies. The 'conclusion' paragraph is not the time to introduce any new themes. However, not to present a concise, summary comment would be a real error of judgement.

Writing and improving your Personal Statement

In formulating the contents of each of the key sections (introduction; main body; conclusion) of your Personal Statement, it is important that you focus upon the following questions:

- Does each of your sections, **especially the introduction,** and your Personal Statement as a whole have **real impact upon the reader?**

- Is the punctuation correct?

- Is the flow of your language appealing, non-repetitive and easy to follow?

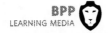

- Is there a logical and coherent balance to the Personal Statement?

- Are all your statements absolutely honest and accurate? Remember! Anything you refer to in your Personal Statement may be the subject of questions at any subsequent interviews. Admissions tutors are very skilled at identifying situations where candidates have made exaggerated claims!

- Will the reader conclude that you are indeed 'special'? Is it truly about you?

And finally:

- **Have you concentrated on justifying and substantiating your comments?**

The admissions tutors will consider everything that you include in your Personal Statement to help them decide whether or not to offer you the opportunity to study Medicine at their university. It is not enough to write, for example: *'I want to study Medicine because Biology is my strongest subject, academically.'* To excel in a specific academic subject is simply not sufficient justification for seeking to make a career within medicine and all that it entails.

Look again at this statement from the quotations presented earlier in Chapter 3:

> *'I find it hard to look back and capture what initially inspired me to take up medicine, but I think that my aspirations are still the same. Medicine is a "way of life" and combines that rather nebulous feeling of wanting to help and care with the more exact principles of science and logical thought.'*

This writer provides clear evidence that it was the combination of their joy in scientific intellectual stimulation **and** the opportunity to reach out and support others that inspired them to study Medicine and develop a medical career.

You must maintain your own focus upon justifying and substantiating your comments throughout your entire Personal Statement.

KEY POINTS

- You need time to write your Personal Statement, do not rush.

- Prepare a first draft, containing an introduction, a main body and a conclusion.

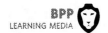

Chapter 6

From 'Draft' to 'Refined': Enhancing your Personal Statement

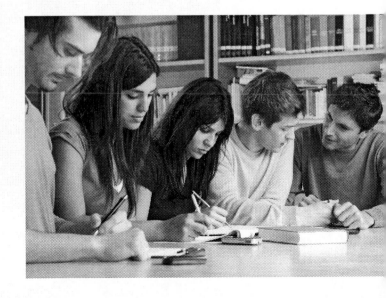

From 'Draft' to 'Refined': Enhancing your Personal Statement

One way by which we can illustrate the importance of focusing on the key principles which govern the preparation of an effective, compelling Personal Statement is to consider a fictitious example, initially in its first 'draft' form, and then looking at it after some refinement. The critique which follows should not be interpreted as 'definitive', or 'state of the art'. And certainly, there is no such thing as the perfect Personal Statement. However, we hope that by using this scenario – moving from a 'draft' to a 'refined' version – we can bring the whole process to life!

Fictitious Personal Statement: 'Draft' version

I have always been fascinated by medicine so I would really like the chance to study it at university. My father and grandfather are both respected doctors and my ambition is to hold a similarly highly regarded position in the community.

I have thoroughly enjoyed studying A levels in Biology, Physics and Chemistry and I also enjoy reading other books about developments in science and I believe I will enjoy studying medicine at University. To explore the subject further I have been to the Medlink conference at Manchester University and Medsim at Nottingham University in 2011.

I have also taken on some work experience in a range of medical areas. I started in 2010 working at Hope House near Reading, which is a residential school for disabled children. I worked there every Wednesday and Saturday afternoon for two years during term-time. Last summer, I went with a group to Ireland for a week to work in a hospice as a volunteer looking after some of the patients there. This was a very demanding experience but it did not discourage me, rather it was one of the most amazing experiences of my life and I plan to return next year. I have also

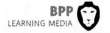

recently started a permanent position as a ward volunteer at Reading District General Hospital. I have also discussed my future career with family members who work in medicine, and I am confident that I am well suited to this career.

I am a keen member of the school science club and I am also captain of the football team, which has won several local tournaments. Playing football and supporting my favourite team, Arsenal, at matches both home and away has given me the chance to meet new people and develop skills in team-working and leadership. I have also been involved in other extra-curricular activities through completing the Duke of Edinbrugh Silver Award. I am also a senior prefect. Art is another hobby of mine, and I like to visit various art galleries in my holidays. I love travelling and I have been to Canada, the USA, France, Italy and Spain. For this reason, I jumped at the chance of a gap year, and I will be working in Britain for six months before I set off travelling.

Character count: 2,111

Fictitious Personal Statement: 'Refined' version

A career in medicine appeals to me as it combines my enjoyment of science with my desire to contribute towards improving the health and wellbeing of people. As several of my relatives are doctors I have benefited from discussions with them about the realities of a medical career, highlighting both the challenges and the rewards.

At school I have found the practical elements of my science subjects particularly fascinating; for example, learning how to use new equipment and materials during experiments. Within Biology I have especially enjoyed learning about the functions of the human body and how different organs behave in health and in disease. Keeping up to date with advances and breakthroughs in medical science is another keen interest of mine, and I regularly read journals such as New Scientist and the BMJ. As a member of the school science club I always look forward to the opportunity to discuss relevant current issues. For example, we had a lively debate about the recent MRSA problems and what might be done to improve the situation; and recently, I gave a short presentation on human stem cell cloning. I am really looking forward to learning more about the ethical issues relating to medical advances during my degree course. Attending the Medlink and Medsim conferences was a valuable way to raise my awareness of what training and a career in medicine will involve, including the need for commitment to the continual updating of my skills and knowledge.

A long-term part-time placement at a residential school for disabled children introduced me to the basics of providing personal care and the need for a sensitive and empathetic approach when talking to patients and their families. This was useful experience for a subsequent position at a hospice in Ireland during which my duties were to befriend and chat to elderly patients. Here I learnt from the nurses about issues such as patient confidentiality and autonomy. My time at the hospice was particularly intense as many of the patients were suffering from mental illnesses associated with cancer. However, I felt inspired by the caring approaches shown by the staff and overall the experience reinforced my commitment towards contributing to this field. Recently, I obtained a weekend position as a ward volunteer at my local general hospital. This has been invaluable in giving me an understanding of how a hospital is run and the functions of the different members of a medical team. My duties so far have involved helping to serve meals, assisting with the personal care of the more mobile patients, and helping with clerical duties in the ward reception area.

In my leisure time I enjoy sport, particularly tennis and football. Captaining my school football team, which has won several local tournaments, has hugely helped me in developing strengths in leadership and teamwork. Completing the Duke of Edinburgh Silver Award gave me the opportunity to learn a range of new

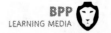

skills, including playing the piano and organising fund raising events. As a senior prefect I am responsible for organising the duties of other prefects; I also assist teachers in supervising lower school pupils at mealtimes and break times. My gap year – during which I intend to travel around South East Asia – will help equip me to live independently and prepare me for the transition between home and university life. Working in a supermarket for six months before leaving will enable me to save the money required and I am confident that a year out of education will be a maturing experience for me.

In conclusion, I am a self-motivated, enthusiastic and determined student who enjoys close interaction with people. I feel prepared for the demands and challenges that a medical career entails. I look forward to the opportunity to read Medicine, in order both to fulfil my ambition of becoming a doctor and to serve the community.

Character count: 3,888

Moving from 'Draft' to 'Refined': Improving your Personal Statement

The following analysis aims to help you to create an engaging Personal Statement by looking at ways the above 'draft' statement was refined. By considering the 'draft' and 'refined' paragraphs side by side, important principles can be highlighted.

Paragraph one: Draft

'I have always been fascinated by medicine so I would really like the chance to study it at university. My father and grandfather are both respected doctors and my ambition is to hold a similarly highly regarded position in the community.'

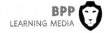

Paragraph one: Refined

'A career in medicine appeals to me as it combines my enjoyment of science with my desire to contribute towards improving the health and wellbeing of people. As several of my relatives are doctors, I have benefited from discussions with them about the realities of a medical career, highlighting both the challenges and the rewards.'

Paragraph one: Draft

The opening sentence is not particularly attention grabbing and does not give the admissions tutors any information beyond that the applicant wants to study Medicine; the admissions panel will have assumed this to be the case anyway. *'I would really like the chance'* is not language depicting a passionate interest in a subject area.

Beware of claiming to have *'always'* been interested in medicine. Even if you did want to be a doctor at the age of three, you would not at that point have had the ability to make an informed decision on the subject. It can sound naïve to imply that you are applying to study a subject because it was your childhood dream. The tutors are looking to see if your choice is based upon careful, mature consideration.

The use of the phrase *'my ambition is to hold a … highly regarded position in the community'* smacks somewhat of a self-seeking motivation. Remember that having a relative or family friend in the medical profession does not in itself improve the applicant's chances of gaining an interview. **If the applicant feels they have benefited from having frequent contact with a practising doctor, it is important that they show they have made use of this opportunity to learn more about the medical career.**

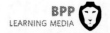

Paragraph one: Refined

By beginning the Personal Statement with a clear and logical explanation of their reason for applying, the candidate now makes a bold and engaging opening sentence and also indicates that they have considered their career choices carefully. This paragraph, therefore, really has become an 'introduction' to the rest of the Personal Statement.

The influence of family members who are doctors is discussed and the applicant refers to the value gained from this personal contact. This does suggest that they are well informed about life as a doctor and therefore may well be the type of person to make the most of opportunities around them.

Paragraph two: Draft

'I have thoroughly enjoyed studying A levels in Biology, Physics and Chemistry and I also enjoy reading other books about developments in science and I believe I will enjoy studying medicine at University. To explore the subject further I have been to the Medlink conference at Manchester University and Medsim at Nottingham University in 2011.'

Paragraph two: Refined

'At school I have found the practical elements of my science subjects particularly fascinating; for example, learning how to use new equipment and materials during experiments. Within Biology I have especially enjoyed learning about the functions of the human body and how different organs behave in health and in disease. Keeping up to date with advances and breakthroughs in medical science is another keen interest of mine, and I regularly read journals such as New Scientist and the BMJ. As a member of the school science club I always look forward to the opportunity to discuss relevant current issues. For example, we had a lively

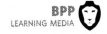

> *debate about the recent MRSA problems and what might be done to improve the situation; and recently, I gave a short presentation on human stem cell cloning. I am really looking forward to learning more about the ethical issues relating to medical advances during my degree course. Attending the Medlink and Medsim conferences was a valuable way to raise my awareness of what training and a career in medicine will involve, including the need for commitment to the continual updating of my skills and knowledge.'*

Paragraph two: Draft

Describing the A level subjects you are studying, information which is picked up elsewhere on your application, simply wastes valuable word space. Although the applicant asserts that they enjoy science, no specific examples are presented to support that comment.

Always ensure that you assign a capital letter to the name of the university course. However, 'university' when used in the general way carries no capital letter. So, *'studying medicine at University'* should read *'studying Medicine at university'*. (Note: It is appropriate for the candidate to provide the capital letters in the specific phrases *'Manchester University'* and *'Nottingham University.'*)

The tone of the paragraph is not enthusiastic: for example, the phrase *'I believe I will enjoy studying medicine at University'* lacks conviction. Remember also that the majority of your fellow applicants will have taken similar subjects at A level and will be predicted similar grades. Coming early in the 'main body' of the Personal Statement, this paragraph provides your opportunity to describe what particularly enthuses **you** and what **you** especially enjoy about the learning process. The admissions tutors will be looking for people who are enthusiastic about the prospect of studying Medicine at their university for several years, as well as looking forward to practising as a doctor later. Although the applicant writes that they like books relating to science, not a single example is cited.

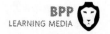

The applicant then states that they have attended Medsim and Medlink conferences but does not explain what they learnt or gained from the experience. Again, remember that many of your fellow applicants will have attended similar conferences; it is up to you to show how this experience has made you a stronger candidate. It is also important not to waste your word limit giving too much irrelevant detail. For example, there is no real need to refer to the location of the conferences you have attended.

Some of the phrases are repetitive: the word 'I' is used five times in less than five lines of text; the words 'enjoyed' and 'enjoy' three times.

Overall, this paragraph adds very little to the Personal Statement and misses an opportunity to show how the applicant has prepared themselves for the academic rigour required in studying for a medical degree.

Paragraph two: Refined

This version provides much greater detail about what the applicant has learnt from their academic experience over the last couple of years. **By describing elements of the subjects which they enjoy, the candidate now highlights their skills in, and their enthusiasm for, practical aspects of science** as well as demonstrating an awareness of how their A level subjects have helped them in preparation for degree level study.

By referring to specific relevant journals and current issues in medicine, the applicant now shows that they are reading outside the school curriculum and provides examples of specific educational areas of interest; their Personal Statement now demonstrates that they have invested some of their own time in support of their commitment to studying Medicine.

Describing what has been gained from the Medlink and Medsim conferences has the same impact. The statements regarding the science club have been moved to this paragraph as they

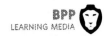

read more fluently and relevantly: they provide good evidence that the candidate has gained valuable experience in broader academic skills, such as conducting self-directed research and in preparing and delivering presentations.

(But remember: referring to, for example, the *BMJ*, provides an open invitation to any interviewer to ask you questions such as 'Tell me about a recent article you have read which has impressed you in some way'. So, make sure you mean exactly what you say in your Personal Statement – and that you do your preparation for interview in that light!)

Paragraph three: Draft

'I have also taken on some work experience in a range of medical areas. I started in 2010 working at Hope House near Reading, which is a residential school for disabled children. I worked there every Wednesday and Saturday afternoon for two years during term-time. Last summer, I went with a group to Ireland for a week to work in a hospice as a volunteer looking after some of the patients there. This was a very demanding experience but it did not discourage me, rather it was one of the most amazing experiences of my life and I plan to return next year. I have also recently started a permanent position as a ward volunteer at Reading District General Hospital. I have also discussed my future career with family members who work in medicine, and I am confident that I am well suited to this career.'

Paragraph three: Refined

'A long-term part-time placement at a residential school for disabled children introduced me to the basics of providing personal care and the need for a sensitive and empathetic approach when talking to patients and their families. This was useful experience for a subsequent position at a hospice in Ireland during which my

---

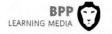

duties were to befriend and chat to elderly patients. Here I learnt from the nurses about issues such as patient confidentiality and autonomy. My time at the hospice was particularly intense as many of the patients were suffering from mental illnesses associated with cancer. However, I felt inspired by the caring approaches shown by the staff and overall the experience reinforced my commitment towards contributing to this field. Recently, I obtained a weekend position as a ward volunteer at my local general hospital. This has been invaluable in giving me an understanding of how a hospital is run and the functions of the different members of a medical team. My duties so far have involved helping to serve meals, assisting with the personal care of the more mobile patients, and helping with clerical duties in the ward reception area.

Paragraph three: Draft

Although the applicant refers to areas of work experience which may well have been extremely helpful when considering whether or not to study Medicine, there is no reflection upon exactly how those experiences helped them to make that decision.

The opening phrase, '*I have also taken on some work experience*' sounds apologetic and wholly lacks enthusiasm. Equally, the '*range of medical areas*' begs the (unanswered) question – exactly which areas? And although describing working in a hospice in Ireland as '*one of the most amazing experiences of my life*' there is absolutely no comment upon why that was the case!

There is also too much space wasted with irrelevant details such as precise times, names and locations. Such details add nothing to the strength of the application. The phrase '*I am confident that I am well suited to this career*' would be better placed within a concluding paragraph.

The phrase '*I have also*' is used three times. The word '*I*' is used nine times!

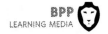

Paragraph three: Refined

The refined version now shows the candidate reflecting upon their work as a volunteer to highlight the experience gained in so many aspects of medical professional work – personal care, empathy, ethical issues, teamwork – and how it has helped them to decide on a career in medicine. Their placement in Ireland clearly was a remarkable experience and served to remind them also of the demands placed upon medical staff when carrying out their day-to-day duties.

Note again:

Because the candidate has introduced topics such as *'patient confidentiality'* and *'autonomy'* it is vital that they obtain a full understanding of their meaning and significance before any interview. By referring to a special interest in the field of mental illness, a similar need for careful interview preparation also applies.

Perhaps the most important aspect of your Personal Statement is the way in which you describe the insights you have gained from your work experience – and indeed how those insights have further encouraged you to pursue a medical career.

Paragraph four: Draft

'I am a keen member of the school science club and I am also captain of the football team, which has won several local tournaments. Playing football and supporting my favourite team, Arsenal, at matches both home and away has given me the chance to meet new people and develop skills in team-working and leadership. I have also been involved in other extra-curricular activities through completing the Duke of Edinbrugh Silver Award. I am also a senior prefect. Art is another hobby of mine, and I like to visit various art galleries in my holidays. I love travelling and I have been to Canada, the USA, France, Italy and Spain. For this reason, I jumped at the chance of a gap year, and I will be working in Britain for six months before I set off travelling.'

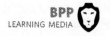

Paragraph four: Refined

'In my leisure time I enjoy sport, particularly tennis and football. Captaining my school football team, which has won several local tournaments, has hugely helped me in developing strengths in leadership and teamwork. Completing the Duke of Edinburgh Silver Award gave me the opportunity to learn a range of new skills, including playing the piano and organising fund raising events. As a senior prefect I am responsible for organising the duties of other prefects; I also assist teachers in supervising lower school pupils at mealtimes and breaktimes. My gap year – during which I intend to travel around South East Asia – will help equip me to live independently and prepare me for the transition between home and university life. Working in a supermarket for six months before leaving will enable me to save the money required and I am confident that a year out of education will be a maturing experience for me.'

Paragraph four: Draft

'Edinbrugh' is an incorrect spelling of the Scottish capital city: the admissions tutors will take a dim view of this example of carelessness! The text reads uninterestingly and the applicant simply lists areas of interest with almost no shades of emphasis or significance – apart from their keenness (*'jumped at'*) to take the opportunity of a year away from academic studies!

The applicant fails entirely to detail how their role as captain of the school football team gives them insights into team-working and leadership, nor do they touch upon the learning value attached to their responsibilities as a senior prefect.

It is hard to see how supporting Arsenal at matches *'home and away'* equips a candidate for medical studies; however, it does indicate how this applicant spends some of their recreational time, inviting a comparison between this and how they invest time in furthering their commitment to a medical career. They

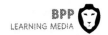

also completely fail to describe the relevance, if any, of their trips to several foreign countries or art galleries.

The word 'I' is used ten times.

Paragraph four: Refined

The points raised about recreational interests and hobbies now focus so much more upon the relevance these pursuits have to the application itself. Details are given as to how being the captain of the football team and involvement in the Duke of Edinburgh Award has helped them become a well-rounded person. Some responsibilities of being a senior prefect are given and the paragraph points to the contributions the student may make to the university community. In their reference to the gap year, they indicate that they have planned a structured year in preparation for life at medical school.

Concluding paragraph: Draft

The 'draft' Personal Statement ends by specifically referring, for the first time, to the theme of the gap year.

The opportunity is not taken to sum up key messages in a final, concluding comment.

Concluding paragraph: Refined

'In conclusion, I am a self-motivated, enthusiastic and determined student who enjoys close interaction with people. I feel prepared for the demands and challenges that a medical career entails. I look forward to the opportunity to read Medicine, in order both to fulfil my ambition of becoming a doctor and to serve the community.'

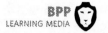

Concluding paragraph: Draft

The candidate has completely failed to take the opportunity to make a final, summary comment. It is as if their entire Personal Statement is left 'hanging in the air'.

Concluding paragraph: Refined

The applicant provides a final summary of their personal qualities aimed at convincing the reader of the sincerity of their application. The closing phrase *'to serve the community'* suggests some understanding of the importance of humility.

KEY POINTS

- The 'Draft' and 'Refined' versions of this fictitious example are presented in order to illustrate the principles underpinning the preparation of a compelling Personal Statement. **Your** Personal Statement must describe **you**; **your** personal qualities, **your** enthusiasms, **your** strengths.

- Make sure the material you present in your Personal Statement really does convince the reader that you have a very good idea of what you are getting into, that studying Medicine is right for you, **and** that you are right for the medical profession.

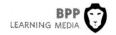

Chapter 7

Personal Statement examples for applying to medical school

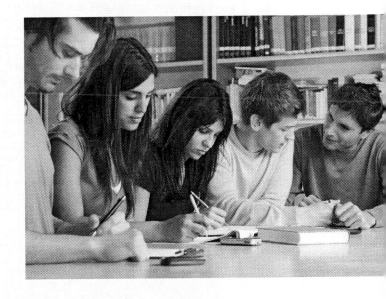

Personal Statement examples for applying to medical school

Undergraduate Personal Statements

Undergraduate Personal Statement 1

My motivation for applying to study Medicine is the desire for a career which will utilise both my empathetic nature and my scientific abilities in helping to improve patients' health and wellbeing. Through work experience placements I have gained a realistic appreciation of both the challenges and the rewards of a career in medicine and I feel I have the qualities and motivation required to be a successful medical student and doctor.

At school I have enjoyed developing practical and evaluative skills in science and have developed a particular interest in human anatomy and physiology in health and disease. I have also been fascinated to learn about the different approach required when treating pregnant women and the adaptations made to clinical procedures when two lives are involved. At university I am looking forward to studying topics such as Neuroscience and Psychology, which interest me as treatment must taken into account the emotional health of the patient, requiring a more holistic perspective. Above all, I am excited about experiencing a wide range of clinical specialties during my studies.

Attendance at a pre-med course gave me an opportunity to hear GPs and other doctors discuss their careers and training, and has helped me understand the different career structures available, as well as highlighting the need for a commitment

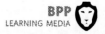

to lifelong learning and professional development. To prepare myself further I will be attending a Medsim course in December. Additionally, my work at a care home for the elderly, providing personal care and befriending residents, has been invaluable in confirming my commitment to a career in healthcare. Through work experience at a GP's surgery I have broadened my understanding of the NHS system, and I made the most of the chance to discuss my future career plans with the GP and the Practice Manager. I was especially interested to observe the GP talking to several patients in their first language, helping them to feel at ease and ensuring they were properly informed about their situation. I also assisted the GP in conducting an ear examination, and in maintaining patient records, ensuring confidentiality was respected at all times. A further placement on a hospital Neuro-Rehabilitation ward saw me shadowing the doctor on his rounds as well as observing and assisting physiotherapists and other allied healthcare workers. Speaking at length to individual patients has helped me to understand the patients' perspective of the health service and through witnessing the doctors dealing with difficult and unco-operative patients I realised the importance of tact, diplomacy and emotional strength.

Visiting and volunteering with children in developing nations, and living in India for several years, has widened my perspective of the world and helped me to foster a flexible and open-minded approach. As a teacher of the Indian dance Bharathanatyam and of primary Mathematics to local children I have strengthened my interpersonal skills, and I have gained confidence through performing at numerous cultural events. Alongside my part-time job at a newsagent's shop and my work as a babysitter, I am also a part-time carer for a family member, which has given

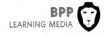

me a valuable insight into the isolation and stress carers can face. Juggling these commitments has ensured I have excellent time management and organisational skills, which will transfer well to life as a medical student. Playing on the school netball team has given me experience of effective teamwork, as well as teaching me how to both win and lose graciously, and I also enjoy trampolining and playing tennis to relax.

In summation, my ambition is to specialise as a plastic surgeon and I look forward to tackling the challenges of studying Medicine and of becoming a skilled and knowledgeable doctor.

Undergraduate Personal Statement 2

As an intelligent, caring and compassionate individual, a career in medicine is suited to me because it incorporates the scientific and intellectual challenges I would require from a profession together with the one-to-one interactions with people which I enjoy. My A level choices have reflected my deep regard for the sciences and through independent learning I have achieved an AS Level in Philosophy and a GSCE in Islamic Studies. A level Chemistry and Biology have furthered my scientific interest and I look forward to learning more about the mechanisms of the human body and also neurology at university. Mathematics has enabled me to develop logical thinking and problem-solving skills which will be beneficial in my future career. Moreover, studying Philosophy has introduced me to ethics, human rights and cultural diversity giving me an appreciation of medical dilemmas eg gene therapy.

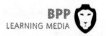

To confirm my interest in Medicine, I spent three days at a health centre shadowing two GPs and sat in on some consultations. After qualifying my goal is to become a GP and I was fascinated to see not only the medical side of a busy surgery and the teamwork involved but also the management and business side of running a busy practice. I also became proficient using Vision, which was their database and consultation software; filing medical histories, making and printing repeat prescriptions and helping with the record keeping of immunisations. I learned that healthcare is not only looking after the physical health of patients but to a certain degree also their mental and emotional health and that GPs are an essential part of the community. Work experience at a bank dealing with customers face to face and on the phone, using basic office equipment, and sitting in on client meetings, reinforced for me that I am suited to a career dealing directly with people in a caring capacity.

As an individual, I have an above average ability to assimilate knowledge and to concentrate for long periods. My extra-curricular activities have included independent study and also taking a responsible role at my Sunday Islamic school which I have attended for the last ten years. Last summer I spent time teaching 10 – 11 year olds numeracy, literacy and science, as well as core Islamic beliefs and Quran reading skills. Following on from this I have been asked to take over another class and I now teach over twenty 10 – 11 year olds Islamic history, Islamic manners and jurisprudence and the Quran, as well as Hadith. The sense of achievement I have experienced has only confirmed that I would like to enter a profession that serves the larger community. While teaching has been demanding it has increased my self esteem and confidence and shown me that I have proficient teaching and communication skills and am able to put across complex

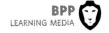

information easily in a friendly way which I believe to be integral to being a successful doctor. I not only interact with the children but also their families and this has developed my interpersonal and teamwork skills. My leadership ability has been enhanced by planning, organising and supervising trips for the children such as visits to the local science museum. Teaching has strengthened personal qualities to manage my time more efficiently, to plan lessons that are interesting and to be perceptive and observant to achieve results, often with a certain amount of wit and humour.

My academic studies and teaching have shown me that as a focused, highly motivated, and determined individual I have the ability to succeed at medical school. My main priority will be concentrating on my studies and I know I have the capacity to apply the skills I have gained to my studies and to commit to a career which will involve continuous learning. I look forward to the challenges and rewards of qualifying and assuming the social responsibility of becoming a GP.

Undergraduate Personal Statement 3

Having travelled extensively through Pakistan, I am fascinated by the link between social, political and economic policies in relation to the health of a nation. I recognised the privilege of having an NHS system in the UK, and this has motivated me towards studying Medicine with the aim of becoming a GP. Contributing to my local community has been a focus for me in my extra-curricular activities and work experience so far, and this is an area I wish to continue developing in. For the past ten months, I have worked within

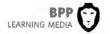

a palliative care environment at Bolton Hospice, gaining first-hand experience helping and interacting with terminally ill patients. I also volunteer as a playschool helper at a local primary school, engaging and entertaining the children in their extra-curricular activities. Additionally, I also work at a local youth club, organising sports tournaments and making youngsters aware of the problems caused by gang culture and drugs. This has been a particularly rewarding experience that has enabled me to gain an insight into many community issues that a GP may face.

Coming from a culture steeped in traditions and customs, I speak both Punjabi and Urdu fluently. For a GP in this community, I believe that I will be able to interact with patients from these ethnic backgrounds with much more empathy and understanding, and gain the trust and rapport required to offer the best level of care for them. I am a confident, enthusiastic and adaptable individual with the ability to lead a team. I have held numerous positions of responsibility at school, including the post of 'Managing Director' of a Young Enterprise business scheme, helping to organise the group and marketing all products and events. In addition, I was elected as a school representative, using this post to act on behalf of the students by liaising with the school authorities, as well as helping with the school's redevelopment plans. This included interviewing prospective applicants to the post of Head Teacher.

Aside from academic study, I enjoy playing football, cricket and rugby. I was awarded the 'Leading Try-Scorer of the Season' trophy for my local rugby club and have also participated in and won numerous football tournaments throughout the borough. Currently, I am working towards my Duke of Edinburgh Bronze Award, a challenge that I am

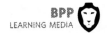

relishing, and which involves taking part in various sports and service provisions. These activities have developed a strong team spirit in me and enhanced my communication skills. I am keen to continue challenging myself in extra-curricular pursuits and am well motivated to embrace all aspects of university life. I am committed to my learning and development, and am already a regular subscriber to medical and science journals such as 'The New Scientist', allowing me to keep up-to-date with recent issues within the medical profession. In particular, I have followed the recent progress in cancer treatment with regard to the drug Herceptin, which has been shown to significantly cut the risk of tumours returning in women with early stage breast cancer. I have also been paying close attention to the advancement of stem-cell research, which is thought to hold huge potential for treating a wide range of diseases and disabilities. This could have a great potential for the development of medicine in the coming years.

To conclude, I believe that I have the academic ability and the community spirit required to be an asset to my chosen university and to become a successful GP.

Undergraduate Personal Statement 4

Throughout my school years I have always wished to pursue a challenging and rewarding profession in which my love of problem-solving and fascination with human physiology and anatomy could be combined with improving the quality of peoples' lives. A career in medicine would allow me to explore the investigative and diagnostic aspects of problem-solving, challenging me mentally and academically while

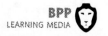

enabling me to work closely with individuals from a wide diversity of cultures.

In order to understand many of the challenges faced by healthcare professionals in both the community, and in hospitals, I sought volunteer placements in a range of different environments. At a busy General Practice I was able to observe General Practitioners during surgeries where, through effective communication with patients, they were able to diagnose and prescribe treatments for a wide range of illnesses and injuries. This emphasis on listening to the patients' needs and concerns was brought home to me on my placement at a nursing home for the elderly. Here I enjoyed being able to interact with the residents, joining in with the games and activities and learning to appreciate the importance of palliative care to ensure the highest possible quality of life. Having sampled how community medicine is practised I arranged further experience in a busy surgical unit at a local hospital. I was privileged to be able to witness intricate surgical procedures such as varicose vein and hernia operations and learned to appreciate the surgeon's skill and expertise, in addition to their level of commitment, integrity and compassion. On one occasion, while a patient was undergoing a surgical procedure under local anaesthetic I was able to talk to him, remaining calm, reassuring and empathetic while the operation was carried out. I also spent time in the Accident and Emergency department and saw how vital communication and teamwork is in making the correct diagnosis and carrying out sometimes life-saving procedures under stressful conditions. Through these placements I gained a valuable insight into the rigorous workload demanded of doctors and observed how members of the healthcare teams work closely together, communicating with patients and their families in decisions regarding their

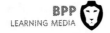

treatment and care. These experiences have helped me to make an informed decision about my future career and have further reinforced my aspiration to study Medicine with the hope of ultimately specialising in surgery or as an Accident and Emergency consultant.

I enjoy new challenges and responsibilities so I was delighted to take part in a biology conservation programme in Honduras where I assisted a team of scientists as we trekked over difficult terrain in order to collect data on a range of endangered species of birds and invertebrates. I particularly enjoyed being able to stretch my communication skills as I was the only member of the group who could speak Spanish, enabling me to make friends with local people and learn more about their culture. The difference in living standards and access to healthcare has been made more apparent to me as I have travelled and this is one issue that I feel strongly about, particularly the ethics regarding the welfare of vulnerable populations of people in poverty, or war stricken regions of the world. Additionally, keeping fit is important to me and I enjoy playing tennis for my school first team and at my local tennis club where I help to coach younger players and encourage friendly tournaments.

To summarise, I know that medicine is a lengthy and demanding career but as an outgoing, hard-working and caring person I know it is the right career choice for me and I look forward to the challenges ahead with the conviction that I can make a positive contribution to the field of medicine.

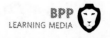

Undergraduate Personal Statement 5

In pursuing a career in medicine I am looking forward to utilising my scientific skills and knowledge within a varied and stimulating profession in which I will have the opportunity to make a real difference to the wellbeing of people from all sectors of society. As a sufferer of chronic nephrotic syndrome myself, I have developed a fascination with the functions of the human anatomy and physiology, and I feel my experience of the patient's perspective will be of great benefit in informing my studies and clinical practice. At university I look forward to studying the science of the human body in health and disease in great detail, and to acquiring the clinical and diagnostic skills required of a successful leader of a medical team.

In my free time I enjoy updating my knowledge through journals such as Student BMJ and recently I have followed the story of patients being cured of cancer after treatment involving genetic modification in the USA with great interest. During my studies I have also been fascinated to learn about the discovery and early use of penicillin and antibiotics in medicine and the scepticism with which such breakthroughs are sometimes initially treated. I am keen to discuss issues such as these, and to speculate on the ways in which medicine will evolve during my own career, with like-minded students at university.

My commitment to becoming a doctor has been strengthened by a range of work experience placements, beginning with a week at a GP surgery in 2010. Through helping the staff with cleaning, typing and paperwork I was able to learn about the running of the practice and develop my communication skills while dealing with patients and their families. This year I have spent a further two weeks at a GP surgery

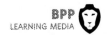

and one week at an out of hours medical centre, assisting staff with administrative work and observing the doctors attending calls. This has broadened my understanding of how the NHS is run and of the different functions of various healthcare professionals. I was especially interested to witness the unique role that a GP can play in the community, offering support with social issues such as contraception and unwanted pregnancies. During the course of my voluntary work I have also noticed the importance of strong and clear communication between the different professionals as well as the need to ensure patients' rights are maintained when dealing with confidential medical records. In October this year I will be spending a week volunteering at a hospital in Birmingham, which will give me further opportunity to learn from practising doctors and prepare myself for entering this career. At present I also have an ongoing role as a volunteer assistant at a residential home for the elderly. This involves befriending the residents and providing personal care, allowing me to hone my listening and interpersonal skills with older people.

As school cricket captain and coach I have developed my leadership skills alongside my cricket technique and I enjoy encouraging the younger students to improve. Through my roles as Head of House and an ICT tutor I have enjoyed contributing to the school community and I look forward to a similar level of involvement in student life at university. Having studied Business at school I have enjoyed making use of my expertise in setting up a small internet retail business with a friend, which takes up much of my free time.

Since the age of eleven I have lived in the UK without my parents, using my determination and self-motivation to

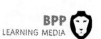

overcome the language barrier and other setbacks. This has helped me to develop an independent and mature approach that will serve me well as I make the transition to university life. My ambition for the future is to serve the community as a GP and I am confident that I have the personal qualities to achieve this goal.

Undergraduate Personal Statement 6

My interest in Medicine originates from a strong academic background complemented by pertinent extra-curricular study and relevant work experience. I have a high regard for the medical profession from personal observation following a close relative's ongoing serious illness and also through my work in hospitals. Having always been fascinated by science, I believe Medicine to be its ultimate application. I am particularly excited about studying pathology, oncology, the human immune system, genetics and biochemistry. After qualifying, I am exploring the option of working as a doctor in the RAF.

Alongside Biology, which has been an introduction to the workings of the human body, studying Chemistry has improved my experimental and analytical skills whereas Mathematics and Geography have enhanced my logical thinking and problem-solving abilities which are relevant to the practice of modern medicine. Studying for the Maryvale Diploma in religious studies places a large emphasis on medical ethics and the questions posed by such cases as Terri Schiavo's. Is a person in a vegetative coma still alive? Should courts decide the fate of a patient? Completing the online course MED-IC has also provided me a valuable insight into Cardiology.

I have spent 100 hours undertaking voluntary work (mainly involving administrative work such as filing, answering phones and booking in patients) and three weeks' work experience at the same hospital shadowing consultants. Although I observed different departments, mainly I was based in the Radiology department where I saw numerous X-rays, ultrasounds and barium enemas. As well as gaining knowledge in these fields I also witnessed the use and benefits of imaging technology such as MRI, dual energy X-rays and CAT scans. I saw the importance of communication and teamwork both in treating patients and between the different departments. Furthermore, at half-term, I have a week's work experience arranged at a local GP surgery. Other relevant experience includes attending the Medsim 2011 course at Nottingham. Seeing the workings of busy hospitals and questioning qualified doctors and lecturers has confirmed I have the ability, confidence and stamina required to complete my training. It has shown me that I'm not interested in a 9 – 5 job and that I am willing to work hard to qualify to achieve a career which requires lifelong commitment. From wider reading I know that medicine is constantly changing with breakthroughs and advances and I have a thirst for knowledge and understanding that will stand me in good stead throughout my career.

At school, as a member of the School Council, and as Treasurer in Year 11, discussing student issues has enhanced my communicative abilities. Working towards the Gold Duke of Edinburgh Award has taught me teamwork, organisational and planning skills. It has also been personally rewarding to be part of my school mentoring scheme. Fully understanding

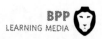

the importance of academic success, I am able to motivate and impart information in a friendly way to younger children. Consequently, I have many transferable skills to apply to my studies together with excellent IT skills. In my spare time I enjoy playing competitive cricket and keep fit and healthy as a member of a local gym and swimming pool. Continuing with my interests will help to offset the pressures and stresses inevitable with my course.

In studying Medicine, I am looking forward to acquiring the scientific knowledge and clinical skills necessary to enable me to diagnose, treat and manage the care of patients. I aim to be fully committed to a profession where continued professional development is integral. In fully researching my medical career, I believe I have the personal qualities and determination to succeed both in my studies and future working life.

Undergraduate Personal Statement 7

Medicine appeals to me as I wish to combine my interest in human anatomy and the interconnecting systems of the body with my desire to help improve people's health in a challenging and hands-on career.

Learning about cardiovascular fitness in PE has been an informative supplement to my science subjects, and I was fascinated by the complexities of the heart after dissecting one in Biology. I am looking forward to studying the cardiovascular system further at university, and also to the dissections as I am a very practical person. I also keep up-to-date with advances and controversies in medicine

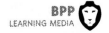

through newspapers and medical literature. Recently I have followed the issue of target times, which I feel may be counterproductive in putting too much pressure on the doctor and possibly resulting in incorrect diagnoses.

During work experience at a GP clinic I carried out administrative tasks on the computer and made use of my opportunity to learn about the running of the clinic and the typical daily workload of a GP. At another clinic I have a regular position transferring records to the computer system. This has developed my IT proficiency as well as allowing me to learn from the range of health professionals using the clinic. Furthermore, at a hospital I volunteer on the trolley rounds selling newspapers and refreshments. This has given me a great deal of contact with patients and has helped me to see their perspective of the hospital experience. I have also learnt how the hospital operates and have particularly noticed the emphasis on teamwork. Volunteering at a nursing home has improved my interpersonal skills as I feed, talk to and provide comfort for the residents. Attending Medsim and Medlink conferences has taught me about the training structure and I enjoyed the practical tasks such as succouring and taking blood pressure. I also have first aid training which has given me some basic medical knowledge.

As a Prefect and Form Captain I set a good example for others and assist the teachers in the smooth running of the school. Taking part in team building exercises at school I learnt skills put to use during my Duke of Edinburgh expeditions. Here I also got to demonstrate leadership and oral communication, supporting and motivating the team when I was leading the group. On the Vinspired programme I have completed over 100 hours of service, organising conferences, coaching PE classes and taking part in the Olympic parade. Completing the Community Sports Leader Award was rewarding, teaching children sports and using my initiative to take control of sometimes difficult situations.

As a competitive sportsman I have helped organise inter-school sports competitions, as well as larger events at Sports Centres. In cricket I am a leg spin bowler and 5th batsman for a club in the East Anglian Premier Cricket League. In tennis I came second in a recent school tournament and I also enjoy practising golf weekly, in which I have a handicap of 19. These achievements have taught me the value of persistence and hard work in achieving goals, and I intend to join the university's teams. Furthermore, DJing provides me with a balance to my academic and sporting commitments. I enjoy garage, hip hop and R'n'B, and have performed a half-hour DJ set on FM 103 Horizon, which involved working under great pressure.

In conclusion, I am a highly motivated and well-balanced student, committed to becoming a doctor and eventually a Cardiologist, and I feel that I have the qualities required to meet the challenges of studying and working in Medicine.

Undergraduate Personal Statement 8

My desire for an academically stimulating career through which I can help to make a positive difference to people's quality of life has motivated me to apply for Medicine. This has been reinforced by extensive work experience in a range of healthcare environments which has confirmed my

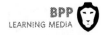

dedication to pursuing this career. Through my schoolwork I have developed a proven ability to manage my time and resources efficiently to meet tight deadlines, and to maintain a consistently high standard over several years. Knowing that Medicine is highly demanding I have researched it thoroughly and, as a naturally positive person with a sense of humour and a wide range of non-academic pursuits, I feel I have the coping strategies necessary to deal with the pressures of a medical degree and career.

I have visited departments including Accident and Emergency, Cardiology and a Diabetes Clinic, learning about the structure of the hospital and the complementary roles played by different members of the team. Attending sessions of Breastfeeding and Child Immunisation Clinics highlighted the importance of prevention as part of successful healthcare provision, and also added to my awareness of the difficult and controversial issues within modern medicine. I have also spent time shadowing a Physiologist, a Cardiologist, and a Community Paediatrician attending child development assessments. I made use of the opportunity to learn as much as possible about a medical career and observed the need for empathy, stamina and dedication across all areas. Having also spent time in a Libyan hospital, at a Burns Clinic for outpatients, I have been able to compare the different health systems and appreciate what the NHS has to offer.

At school I was a senior member of the Health Awareness Committee, organising and delivering campaigns in healthy eating and smoking awareness. This involved liaising with members of the team, and motivating and supporting others. At the Autism Unit I helped support children with autism and Asperger's syndrome to achieve their best, acted as a mentor in the 'buddy system' and worked as a classroom

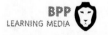

assistant with first year pupils. Doing regular babysitting jobs has shown me the importance of being patient and creative when dealing with children; my first aid skills also prove useful when dealing with minor injuries. During my gap year I am volunteering at a nursing home where I am learning about the particular needs of the elderly and experiencing hands-on primary care. I will also be continuing my work as a Samaritan. There I take calls from severely troubled people and have received training in the listening skills and non-judgmental manner which are required to help the callers. This work appeals to my empathetic nature and has given me an insight into mental health problems. In these environments, as well as in a charity shop, I am developing excellent communication and interpersonal skills with a diversity of patients, families, customers and colleagues.

At school I was on the newspaper team, writing articles and helping to sell issues. This provided a great creative outlet and I am continuing to write short stories and poetry. When the Scottish weather permits I enjoy hill-walking and landscape photography. Developing my images using Photoshop software I also create avatars, wallpapers, and music videos. I also play in a local netball club and go jogging most weekends, and I am currently teaching myself Arabic dancing. In an effort to expand my communicative potential and to prepare myself for my continental travels I am currently learning French.

I am fully committed to my aim of becoming a successful doctor providing the best possible care for my patients and I believe I have the skills and motivation to achieve my goals.

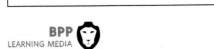

Undergraduate Personal Statement 9

My interest in Medicine began on a visit to India, during which I witnessed the disabilities and deaths that result from preventable diseases such as cholera and malaria. My own cousin suffers from severe sensory neural hearing loss as a result of his mother contracting rubella during her first trimester. The fact that in the UK this could have been prevented by a routine vaccination is a stark illustration of the importance of medical care.

I have a passion for science, and for its potential to contribute positively to people's lives, and this is reflected in my school learning. There I thoroughly enjoyed my Chemistry A level, particularly the group research and practical experiments, and I found learning about human anatomy and physiology in Biology highly interesting. I am looking forward to studying clinical procedures at university and acquiring sufficient knowledge to give accurate diagnoses and prescriptions. I am passionate about raising awareness of health issues and am currently setting up diabetes awareness sessions at local supermarkets. I also work with Directorate of Organ Donation & Transplantation to raise awareness of donor cards amongst the Asian community.

During work experience in a postnatal unit I assisted the midwifery team in the care of the babies, and observed premature babies being cared for in incubators. Contributing to staff meetings in which patients' progress was discussed, I learnt about a variety of issues affecting the hospital. Recently, I completed a clinical attachment at Harefield Hospital with a Consultant Audiological Physician, a fascinating experience from which I learnt a great deal. Attending multidisciplinary meetings I noticed how professionals from different specialties came together to

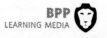

form a team to give the best possible care. I also attended a clinic for babies and children undergoing chemotherapy for life threatening cancers. This gave me some appreciation of working in a sensitive atmosphere with terminally ill children and distraught parents, requiring a tactful and compassionate manner.

For the past eighteen months I have worked part-time at a home for people with severe learning and physical disabilities. This has been extremely rewarding working in a team of carers to deliver all aspects of personal care, including manual handling using hoists and administration of daily drugs. On night shifts I have the responsibility of being shift leader, requiring me to show leadership, initiative and a calm but efficient response to any problems. I use good verbal communication to ensure the staff works together and to give a precise verbal handover at the end of a shift. Monitoring residents to ensure the correct drugs and tests are given has required great attention to detail, and through maintaining accurate reports I have developed clear written communication and good organisational skills.

In my year out I will be working with children and disabled adults in the UK, as well as travelling to Costa Rica to work for the charity 'School 2 Escuela'. As school Charity Rep I am involved in fundraising events for breast cancer and heart disease charities. I enjoy sports and captained the athletics team for several years, organising events and supporting encouraging team members. I also enjoy performing on stage and recently played the lead role in a school production. My participation on the public speaking team has boosted my confidence in presenting and justifying my views and I also enjoy working on the college newsletter.

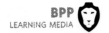

In the long term I hope to specialise in Dermatology and to be able to deliver the best possible healthcare to the community. I am totally committed to becoming a doctor and I feel that I have the skills and motivation to succeed at university and in my future career.

Undergraduate Personal Statement 10

The premature birth of my sister when I was 12 was pivotal in my decision to study Medicine as I wish to be able to provide the same treatment and support to others as was offered to my family. At school I have enjoyed my A level studies and particularly the role of Physics in Medicine, such as in ECHO and MRI technology. Witnessing these procedures while on work experience has allowed me to marry my theoretical knowledge with first-hand observations. Reading 'New Scientist' and other related literature, I have explored some of the controversies of modern Medicine.

At Bristol Royal Infirmary I shadowed House Officers and Registrars in Cardiac and Respiratory Medicine. Attending outpatient clinics, observing bronchoscopies and angiographies, and observing MRIs and ECHOs, I had an insight into some specialist areas. Following this I was offered a paid job in the outpatients reception, where I still work. This has allowed me to learn a great deal about the structure of a hospital, and to see the significance of teamwork between all members of staff. The importance of trust between patient and doctor, and the role of open communication and active listening in achieving this, has also been demonstrated. I have made full use of the opportunity to learn about the profession from doctors and

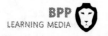

medical students I have worked alongside. I have recently been asked to assist a Research Fellow in a long-term project monitoring the first ever patients to receive septal ablation treatment for hypertrophic cardiomyopathy. This is ongoing research which I am working hard on, and which is likely to result in publication.

As a St John Ambulance Volunteer I trained in first aid and have some appreciation of the need for calm and efficiency when dealing with emergencies. I have also gained the UK Sports Coach Qualification for my work with the Horizon Sports Club, a branch of Special Olympics UK. This involves teaching, supporting and motivating children with autism and severe physical disabilities in football. This has included one-to-one coaching and some work alongside the Senior Coach, vastly improving my confidence in communicating with people of all ages and abilities. It is an exceptionally rewarding experience and has illustrated the importance of continued psychological support as part of a successful treatment package. I have also volunteered in helping nurses and befriending patients at Wycombe Hospital, which has allowed me to see the hospital from a patient's perspective.

At school I was one of a team of senior prefects, supervising my own group of regular prefects and helping staff with the smooth running of the school. Organising and delivering assemblies in front of a large audience has developed my presentation and organisation skills and I also enjoy mentoring younger pupils in Physics and Chemistry. To unwind from my studies and responsibilities I enjoy performing in the orchestra, jazz band and saxophone quartet, having taught myself saxophone, guitar and piano. I am also Head of Boarding, supporting other pupils, and

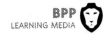

as a boarder myself I have developed the independence and self-motivation associated with living away from home. This will be useful when I start at university and I intend to make the most of the facilities by continuing my musical hobbies and my enjoyment of tennis, as well as taking up rowing.

In the long term I aim to become a hospital consultant and possibly a surgeon. Having researched my career choice thoroughly I feel I have the skills and motivation to be a success in this. I am fully committed to becoming a doctor and I look forward to working as part of a team applying science and compassion to save and sustain lives.

Undergraduate Personal Statement 11

A career in Medicine offers unique challenges and responsibilities alongside significant scope for personal and professional development in a variety of fields. As an outgoing, hard-working and enthusiastic student I am also attracted to the ever-evolving nature of medical science and the opportunity to play a positive role in people's lives.

Attendance at a Medsim conference, during which I witnessed surgery and practised my own manual skills using real medical tools and equipment, taught me about the different specialties available within medicine and about the different skills which are required by these. I was also lucky enough to visit St Thomas' operating theatre on a school trip to London. While touring the 19th century hospital I was fascinated to learn about the changing role of medicine within society, as well as the technological

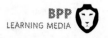

advances which have been made. Since this trip I have read several books on current controversial developments such as the increasing use of computer technology in diagnosis and in surgery. Studying an Open University course on 'Molecules, Medicines and Drugs' has allowed me to explore the development of drugs and their use in curing illnesses and relieving pain. The course is equivalent to ten credits at undergraduate level and has introduced me to self-directed study and time management. At school I have worked hard to achieve high grades, including receiving the Year Prize for Chemistry and Biology last year, and I intend to bring the same level of commitment to my higher level studies.

A week long work observation placement at a general hospital gave me the opportunity to observe spinal surgery, ECG scans and endoscopies, as well as outpatients' clinics for stroke victims. This equipped me with a valuable insight into the organisation of a hospital and a realistic appreciation of the skills required to be a successful doctor and the role played by effective multidisciplinary teamwork in delivering patient care. I have also worked in a pharmacy shop, serving customers and arranging stock, which has introduced me to several common medical conditions and their treatments, and allowed me to develop customer service skills and confidence in oral communication. I am currently taking a gap year, giving me a chance to develop my independence before progressing to university, and have recently begun a voluntary placement in the specialist burns unit at Royal Alexandra Hospital, which is proving an excellent supplement to my previous medical experience. Combining this with voluntary care work with a local project offering practical assistance to young people with learning difficulties has widened my employment experience and I am also

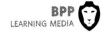

applying for work as a care assistant at a local care home, which I hope will prove a useful learning experience.

At Sixth Form College I enjoyed contributing to the student community as a Student Representative and the Vice President of the Young Muslim Society, both of which have given me experience of co-operating within a team and of expressing and defending my ideas articulately. Completing my Gold Duke of Edinburgh Award, the first person at my college to do so, has given me the chance to develop new skills such as making presentations, conducting research and leading a group. I have also gone from being a beginner to passing Grade 7 in guitar, performing publicly as part of the Award, and I look forward to involving myself in new hobbies and interests at university.

In conclusion, I consider myself to be a well-rounded and dynamic student, with significant relevant experience, and I look forward to the challenges and rewards of life as a medical student.

Undergraduate Personal Statement 12

Studying a degree in Medicine will allow me to explore more deeply my interest in the physiology and anatomy of the human body, and to gain the clinical and diagnostic skills required to make use of this knowledge. Extensive work experience has confirmed my enjoyment of working closely with others and I look forward to being in a position to contribute to improving patients' health.

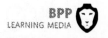

My A levels have given me a basic understanding of the functions and processes of the human body and I am particularly looking forward to studying the digestive system and the role nutrition plays in maintaining good health. The functions of the heart, blood and circulatory system also fascinate me and this interest has been boosted by my experience of shadowing a Consultant Cardiologist. Reading the BMJ online and books such as those of Richard Dawkins and Stephen Hawking has supplemented my schoolwork and introduced me to some of the key controversies and debates within science. At my school's philosophy club I have enjoyed debating issues such as 'God v Science' and I am looking forward to discussing ethical dilemmas within medical practice, such as those associated with human cloning and genetic engineering, with my fellow students at university.

Four weeks' work experience in a large general hospital has given me an appreciation of both the rewards and challenges of a medical career. During my first week I observed staff within several departments and was able to witness MRI scans, endoscopies and CT scans. Shadowing doctors during ward rounds, clinics and departmental meetings has helped me to understand the variety of a doctor's typical workload and highlighted the importance of effective communication and teamwork within and between different departments. Two weeks in Accident and Emergency, observing the treatment of various minor and major injuries, was enlightening and I was lucky enough to be allowed to practise taking patient histories. This gave me the chance to utilise my own communication skills and demonstrated the importance of listening carefully and empathising in order to put the patient at ease. This was followed by a week shadowing a Consultant Cardiologist

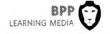

throughout all his duties, from diagnosing and treating patients to completing paperwork and chairing meetings. Shadowing a GP for a further week helped me to make sense of the NHS referral system and I learnt a great deal about the importance of community medicine and the role of nurses and other healthcare professionals within this. For several months I have also volunteered one day a week at a nursing home, giving me further experience of a caring role and introducing me to some of the specific needs of elderly patients. Much of my role here involves chatting to residents and helping them to feel more comfortable; this has given me confidence talking to people from different age groups and social backgrounds.

Through my role as a mentor, assisting younger pupils with literacy and numeracy, I have developed my leadership skills and gained confidence working under my own initiative. These strengths were further utilised during an outdoor adventure course with the YMCA, which involved finding solutions to problems such as crossing a river without getting wet using limited resources. This also helped me to learn how to contribute effectively to a team and communicate disagreement with other team members in a calm and constructive way.

Research into my career options has ensured I am fully aware of both the benefits and difficulties of life as a doctor and I look forward to making the most of the academic, social and sporting opportunities available to me at university.

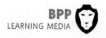

Undergraduate Personal Statement 13

A degree in Medicine will give me the chance to achieve my ambition of pursuing a stimulating and challenging career through which I can make a genuine contribution to people's quality of life. Healthcare work experience and my personal experience as a young carer has given me a rounded understanding of the challenges faced by medical staff, patients and families. Through training as a doctor I hope to have the opportunity to provide treatment and support for patients struggling with lifelong illnesses and disabilities.

In order to learn more about the career structure and options available within medical training I have attended Medlink and Medsim conferences. The importance of effective communication and strong, trust-based teamwork within the clinical environment was highlighted by the simulated emergency scenario and I enjoyed putting my skills to the test. Working at a school for physically and mentally disabled children for two months has given me a fuller appreciation of the wider healthcare system and has introduced me to a range of paediatric conditions and the importance of effective palliative care for people with long-term health problems. This volunteer role has also developed my interpersonal skills and my self-confidence. For the last seven years I have been involved in providing daily personal care for my mother, who suffers from multiple sclerosis. This has given me experience of administering injections, lifting and handling a disabled person and providing emotional, as well as physical support. In order to be able to provide a high level of care I have completed training in first aid and CPR and through attending multiple sclerosis meetings and clinics and reading up on the subject in my spare time I have learnt a great deal about this fascinating area

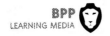

of medicine. Neuroscience, as well as Pharmacology and Pathology, is one of the clinical subjects I am most looking forward to addressing during my degree, particularly as there is still so much to be discovered about how the brain and nervous system. My own reading on these areas of medicine, primarily through first year undergraduate text books, has supplemented the knowledge I have gained through Biology and Chemistry A levels.

At school I am involved in a reading scheme with the primary school, which requires me to spend two periods a week encouraging Year 1 pupils to enjoy reading and other literacy activities. This has widened my experience of working with people of different ages and I have taken pride in seeing the children's confidence develop. Since the age of eight I have competed in local football teams and have represented my school for three years. When playing sport I enjoy the support and camaraderie of being part of a strong team, as well as the opportunity to develop my physical fitness and agility. At present I am taking a gap year in order to develop my life experience. As well as working at a local gift shop, serving customers, ordering stock and arranging displays, I am spending two days a week working at a care home for the elderly. I also intend to complete my 200 hours of community service as a volunteer for the Vinspired programme and I feel this time away from education will allow me to develop my independence and maturity in preparation for the transition to university.

My goal after qualifying is to work towards becoming a Consultant Surgeon specialising in the field of Neuroscience. As a highly motivated, well-rounded and ambitious student with a genuine commitment to a career in medicine, I am confident that I have the qualities to achieve this ambition.

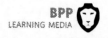

Undergraduate Personal Statement 14

I resolved to study Medicine at university on first encountering topics such as the cause, action, and diagnosis of disease in Biology GCSE. To be in a position to diagnose someone's problems and provide a solution which will cure them or alleviate their pain is my vocation and I have focused throughout the last two years on achieving my best at school and obtaining sufficient experience to fully understand what a medical career involves.

Studying Biology A level and discovering the intricacies of the human body has been captivating for me and I am especially drawn towards the modules on the genetic code and its possible use in medicine. Advances in genetic engineering have the potential to revolutionise clinical practice and I am fascinated by people's varied responses to the emotive issue of its use in reproductive medicine. Discussing such issues within classes has helped me to formulate my own ideas and, during my hospital work experience, I have been interested to find out the views of practising doctors on how they separate their personal views and professional opinions. Through reading the BMJ and New Scientist I am able to keep myself up-to-date with scientific developments and further develop my interest in molecules, cells and disease.

Throughout my A levels I have volunteered weekly at a school for children with learning difficulties, assisting the teachers and classroom support staff. This has enhanced my interpersonal skills, as well as my creativity and empathy when trying to find ways to communicate with the children. As many of the children also have physical disabilities I have learned about the time and effort put in by parents and teachers to meet the children's needs, which will help

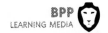

me to relate to carers and families I will meet as a medical student. Last summer I spent a month at a 'hospital' for Lourdes pilgrims, assisting with the visitors' personal care and accompanying them on their outings to the miracle site. As well as furthering my experience of caring, this opened my eyes to the variety of ways people choose to deal with terminal illness and the different things which can bring people comfort. I realised the importance of cultural sensitivity and the difficulties of not imposing my own personal views on those I was caring for. The intensity of this experience, including surviving on less than three hours' sleep a night, and the sense of inspiration and purpose I gained from my team, gave me confidence that I have the stamina to meet the challenge of life as a medical student. As I live in a very remote area I have not had access to a hospital in which to do work experience as I would have liked. However, spending a week shadowing a community nurse, and discussing my future career with her as well as observing her at work, and attending Medlink and Medsim conferences, have gone some way to counter this and I feel I have a good understanding of the structure of medical training and the variety of career options available.

During my gap year I will add to my UK healthcare experience with a six-month medical placement in Pakistan. I expect this work to be tiring and emotionally difficult as many of the patients are from the most deprived areas and cannot afford to pay for treatments. Living away from home for this time will develop my maturity and ensure I am familiar with issues such as managing my time and money, allowing me to concentrate fully on my studies when I begin university. In my free time I have been working towards my Duke of Edinburgh Silver Award which has taught me the importance of practice and persistence, as well as providing experience of working effectively within a team. My work experience has demonstrated the importance of these skills for a doctor and I am confident that, if given the opportunity to study Medicine, I will be able to make good use of these qualities in pursuing my vocation.

Undergraduate Personal Statement 15

The principle elements of medicine which appeal to me are the daily interaction with people of all ages and backgrounds, and the rewarding nature of helping to alleviate their suffering. The essential role of a doctor, particularly a GP, within the community also attracts me to the profession as I feel my interpersonal skills and enjoyment of helping others would make me ideally suited to this role.

My interest in Medicine developed after a careers fair at my school which included a talk by a second year medical student about his experiences at university. Talking to him after his presentation helped me to gain a clear idea of exactly what is required to study at this level and motivated me to continue studying Chemistry, Mathematics and Biology to A level, a decision which has been very rewarding. I have very much enjoyed developing the practical skills associated with these subjects, conducting experiments in order to test a hypothesis and analysing the results, particularly when findings are unexpected. Practical work has also helped me to develop an eye for detail and accuracy. Throughout my time at college I have worked hard to develop my time management, problem-solving and presentation skills. Participating in the science and debating clubs has enhanced my oral communication skills and I am keen to involve

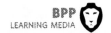

myself in academic societies when at university. During my degree I look forward to taking part in the 'doctor and patient' sessions as I find problem-based learning particularly engaging. I am also keen to experience the wide variety of specialties which university will introduce me to.

Work experience at an NHS dental surgery last year was my introduction to healthcare practice and I enjoyed the high levels of patient interaction which were a constant part of the dentist's role. Reassuring nervous patients, especially children, was rewarding and through working in the reception I gained an understanding of the NHS referral system and the interdisciplinary nature of patient management. Spending a further two weeks shadowing a Paediatrician has helped to confirm my decision to study Medicine. The range of conditions treated fascinated me and I learned about the emotional highs and lows experienced by those working on the children's ward. The importance of sensitive communication skills was clear and I was able to discuss with the Registrar the techniques he used to help patients and their parents deal with their illness. I am currently in the process of arranging further healthcare work experience in order to strengthen my knowledge of the sector prior to studying Medicine.

Working part-time as an assistant at a fast food restaurant has tested my time management and interpersonal skills as I have had to combine employment with studying and have worked with colleagues of all ages and backgrounds. Playing lead roles in several school plays has improved my confidence in performing before a large audience and I also enjoy my role as captain of a local junior rugby team. Having competed at national level in gymnastics I now teach younger gymnasts and am currently undertaking

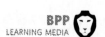

my bronze coaching award. I have also contributed my organisational skills to several fundraising campaigns within my local community, including helping to raise £1,500 through a sponsored walk and £400 via a fashion show at which I supervised the backstage crew. My research into possible careers has shown that strengths in teamwork, communication and leadership are all essential to success as a medical student and doctor and over the last two years I have developed these qualities to a high level. If given the opportunity to study Medicine I will strive to continue to achieve my best in all areas of university life.

Undergraduate Personal Statement 16

My desire to become a doctor has developed from a deeply personal interest in healthcare from a patient's perspective. At the age of 15 I had to leave school early due to ill health; I was under the care of my local hospital for three years and it was during this time that my passion for medicine flourished. Regaining my health required great efforts on my part, and strong support from the medical profession, and the experience taught me greater tolerance, dedication and determination. My ambition is now to become a GP within the community.

At university I am looking forward to learning more about long-term conditions such as hypertension and diabetes and also emergency medicine, as this builds upon what I have already learned from being a first aider. I have fully researched a degree in Medicine and understand the rigours that studying will entail. I have an enquiring mind and

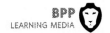

would relish having a career that combined working with people with constant change and continuous learning.

Returning to college to complete my secondary education has been challenging. My life experiences to date have shown me I have the resilience to overcome difficulties which should stand me in good stead during my studies at medical school and in my future career. My studies have given me transferable skills to take with me to university. Studying A level Human Biology has given me an in-depth understanding of the human anatomy and physiological processes and Chemistry has helped develop my analytical and research skills. Environmental Science explores human impact on, and the interactions between, the physical, chemical and biological components of the environment. Consequently my interest has been stimulated to study Physics in my final year.

While medicine is a scientifically based career it requires interpersonal skills and the ability to empathise with people. This approach to a career suits both my skills and character, and I believe that this is the best career for me. I wish my vocation in life to be beneficial to others. To confirm that I am suited to a career in medicine, I work as a volunteer at a care home for the elderly during the holidays and every Saturday during term time. My duties involve supporting and co-operating with the OCT team to promote independent activity and continued healthy brain function in the residents. It has shown me the empathetic side to my nature which means that I can listen to people and their problems with sensitivity and understanding and improve their quality of life. I am also an active member of St John Ambulance where I learnt first aid and regularly attend duties. Both activities have enhanced my interpersonal and communication skills with people at all levels. Acting as a first aider requires me to be articulate and decisive with the adoption of a clear leadership role when serious medical conditions require urgent attention.

In my spare time, I enjoy caving which requires adept teamwork skills to prevent accidents. It is demanding but personally rewarding hobby and appeals to the calm and logical aspects of my personality. It has also taught me coping mechanisms for dealing with stressful situations which I can apply to my future studies. My hobby is collecting antique books, both medical and literary, as I enjoy reading about medical and social history of the time. To widen my experience, I regularly attend talks and debates with well-known authors, scientists and politicians, such as: John Mortimer, Professor Lewis Walport and Michael Howard. At university I would like to continue my interests and possibly try new activities to act as a balance to my studies. As a mature, committed and hard-working individual I am looking forward to the challenges of study and the rewards of my future career.

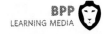

Mature Personal Statements

Mature Personal Statement 1

In training to be a doctor I wish to develop the skills and knowledge to help people during their most vulnerable times. As I am interested in the human aspect of the job, the clinical skills lessons and learning about the psychological aspects of coping with illness are appealing. Since leaving school I have harboured a persistent desire to become a doctor although my career path has taken me in other directions. I feel that I am now in a position to make use of my communication skills, emotional maturity, experience of stressful situations and renewed hunger for learning by committing myself fully to Medicine.

Learning from my GP father about the pros and cons of the job I am entering the profession with a realistic view of the challenges involved. I have recently started a job as a paid part-time theatre assistant which involves waiting with patients before and after theatre, building a rapport with them and monitoring their needs, as well as assisting in manual handling of patients, managing stock levels and cleaning and preparing theatres. This will be a wonderful opportunity to learn more about medicine and to discuss issues with current students and qualified professionals in order to prepare myself fully for my degree. In November I will be assisting my father on a trip to Antarctica during which he will be the expedition doctor. My role will be to help with the manual side of setting up and running the surgery on board the ship.

My career with the Royal Engineers has provided me with a range of skills transferable to a career in medicine. While serving in Kosovo I managed several construction projects in

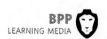

an unstable Serbian-occupied region and executed searches for drugs, bodies and weapons. This required effective communication, working with people who were often in fear of violence and in highly stressful situations. Being in sole charge of difficult situations I have used initiative, ingenuity and problem-solving skills to meet deadlines. Working in a war zone I demonstrated sensitivity and respect for diversity as well as the ability to cope with sleep deprivation and work calmly under pressure. After completing my training I had responsibility for the personal development of over 100 soldiers. I also managed engineering courses and delivered lessons to trainees, as well as my peers and seniors, about balancing resources with maintaining Health and Safety standards. In the army interpersonal skills and cohesive teamwork are emphasised and I have a non-confrontational manner in such situations. While a Police Officer I encountered several difficult situations such as moving deceased bodies, informing relatives and dealing with a sexual assault victim, violent shoplifters and a heroin addict. I feel this has prepared me for the less appealing aspects of medicine.

As a BSAC Sports Diver I enjoyed my position as Chairman of the Eastern Cyprus Sub Aqua Club and have dived around the world. I captained our snowboarding team and am a keen surfer and I intend to participate in corresponding university clubs. As Entertainments Manager of the officers' mess I also organised events such as the summer ball attended by over 600 guests.

In the long term I am interested in the community involvement of being a GP and I feel it would be rewarding to build a rapport with families through the generations. From my career experience of working under pressure, and

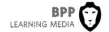

having already developed the support network and outside interests required to maintain a healthy work-life balance, I feel I am well prepared for commencing my medical career. As a mature entrant I have given up my career to focus full-time on getting into Medicine and I feel I have the skills and motivation required to achieve my ambition.

Mature Personal Statement 2

Devoting myself to making a positive contribution to the field of healthcare has been a desire of mine since I was a young child visiting my local GP with my mother. I was enthralled by the doctor's good-hearted nature and commitment to others and my admiration for those in the medical profession has only grown since. However, owing to financial constraints when finishing school and then the raising of a young family it is only now, with my two children now in full-time education, that I can apply myself to becoming a doctor.

When at school I took great pleasure from my Biology A level as I was fascinated by the physiology and workings of the human body, as well as learning about historical breakthroughs in the field of medicine, such as Alexander Fleming's discovery of penicillin. Chemistry improved my research skills and helped fuelled my interest in science at a molecular level, whereas my Physics A level I found often stimulating, helping develop my cognitive thinking skills. I am aware that it has been some time since I finished my school studies and so to rectify this I have been attending night classes in Biology and ICT at a local college to ease

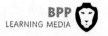

myself back into a learning environment and prepare myself for the rigours of university study.

In preparation for entry into medical school I have recently attended the Medsim course at Nottingham. Meeting doctors and current medical students and hearing them talk of their passion for Medicine, despite the heavy commitment required, only further consolidated my desire to become a doctor myself one day. Moreover, I shadowed doctors at Queen Mary Hospital, Kent, over a period of six weeks this year where I have had the privilege to observe patient treatment and procedures in Paediatrics, Obstetrics and Gynaecology, and Accident and Emergency, being allowed in some cases to assist in history-taking and minor procedures. I was consistently impressed by the focus and effectiveness of the multidisciplinary approach taken to ensure the optimum care for patients and look forward to being a part of such an approach in the future. Additionally, during this last year I have worked part-time as a receptionist at my local GP practice which has been an invaluable experience as I have been exposed to the administrative side of healthcare and interaction with patients. Moreover, for the past five years I have worked part-time at a local supermarket, and despite my part-time status managed to attain the position of shift supervisor. This position entailed the supervising of junior colleagues, delegating of tasks and effective communication skills, all talents which I believe should hold me in good stead for the future.

In my spare time at the weekend I volunteer at a local playgroup for children with learning disabilities where I interact with children suffering from a range of conditions, including autism. This experience has informed my interest in Paediatrics, a field which I can envision myself working within in the future, assessing and treating those with development disorders. I value the importance of a healthy work and leisure balance to relieve stress and in my spare time I enjoy cycling, cooking and spending time with my family. Managing a family and a career has endowed me with excellent time management skills and I look forward to contributing to university life while at medical school; I would be interested in joining a cycling or cookery club or society if one exists on campus.

In closing, I believe that my life experiences, coupled with my commitment and drive to helping others as a doctor, should enable me to perform to my fullest capabilities at medical school as an ideal student.

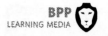

Postgraduate Personal Statements

Postgraduate Personal Statement 1

Medicine offers a varied, challenging and stimulating career, with extensive opportunities for rapid personal and professional development. Extensive work experience has allowed me to make a realistic appraisal of a career in medicine, and I look forward to utilising my passion for scientific knowledge in relieving the pain and suffering of others.

My degree in Human Genetics has equipped me with a strong grounding in cellular and molecular biology, as well as an understanding of the role of genes in different human organisms. I have developed a particular interest in the aspects of genetic research that can be used to identify, and possibly treat or cure, human disease. For my third year project I have therefore chosen to spend time researching the genetic alteration of mice to model various human genetic diseases. The mice are treated with mutagen and those that show phenotypes correlating with those shown by humans with a particular neuromuscular disease are selected and bred from to create an inbred strain of mice. DNA samples are then taken with the final aim of being able to locate the genes responsible for that particular disease and using them in genetic testing or to help find gene-targeted treatments for specific diseases. At university I am looking forward to complementing my understanding of this aspect of medical science with the study of physiology and anatomy and the acquisition of diagnostic and clinical skills.

Shadowing a Consultant Gastroenterologist for two weeks has given me an invaluable insight into the day-to-day work of a successful doctor, sitting in on clinics and

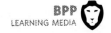

observing several procedures such as colonoscopy, upper GI endoscopy and the endoscopic removal of biopsies. This familiarised me with the techniques used to communicate sensitively with patients and their families, demonstrating the need for patience, empathy and active listening skills. A further week in an Orthopaedic department, shadowing doctors during ward rounds and clinics, has broadened my understanding of the NHS and the functions of each member of a healthcare team. The importance of good communication in creating effective teams was clear. Before my degree I spent a gap year working in the quality assurance department of a pharmaceutical company, cross-referencing internal documents alongside legal requirements to ensure compliance with the strict regulatory requirements enforced on pharmaceutical companies. I was also involved in a range of projects involving the redesign of product packaging and interacted with everybody from shop floor staff to senior management. Since June this year I have been working as a receptionist and administrator at a hospital day surgery. These roles have familiarised me with the medical world and I have enjoyed discussing current issues within the profession, such as the recent modernising of the structure of new doctors' training and the efforts to meet the confines of European working time directives.

Further voluntary work, at a school for children with autism and special educational needs, a youth club for underprivileged teenagers, and an after-school activity club, has allowed me to develop my own communication and interpersonal skills while helping young people to enhance their skills and confidence. In my leisure time I enjoy relaxing through sports such as swimming and ice skating, having completed all National Federation grades. I also play clarinet and piano to a high level and have performed as first clarinet in a local clarinet choir, orchestra and wind band. As a graduate student I have researched my career options thoroughly and am fully committed to the work involved in succeeding in Medicine. I would like to utilise my Genetics degree by practising in a related specialty and I believe I have the skills and motivation to achieve this goal.

Postgraduate Personal Statement 2

Medicine offers a varied and rewarding career which will allow me to apply clinical knowledge to real life situations in order to improve people's health and wellbeing. I am confident that this career path will make the best use of my academic ability, people skills and personal disposition. After completing a degree in Biochemistry last year, and reviewing the career options available to me, I felt drawn to Medicine due to my experience as a part-time ward clerk over the last three years. Interacting with patients and their families gives me a sense of fulfillment and the feeling that, even as a non-medical member of staff, I am able to make a positive difference to people's experience of medical treatment. A period of temporary work in a research laboratory, during which I enjoyed delving deeper into my subject but felt distanced from the ultimate purpose of the research, confirmed for me that patient interaction is essential for me to gain job satisfaction.

My work experience in a number of hospitals and clinics has been an opportunity to fully explore the healthcare profession, from the structure and organisation of the NHS to skills needed within different medical specialties. Last

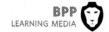

Easter I shadowed a local GP during her rounds and I enjoyed observing her interactions with nurses, pharmacists and carers and the way in which she had integrated herself into the local rural community. The need for doctors to constantly work towards keeping pace with advances within their medical field, and within the profession as a whole, was also made clear as the GP spent a significant portion of her time reading journals and research findings. Following the treatment process, from initial consultation through diagnosis and treatment to follow-up, gave me an insight into the doctor's decision-making process as well as the level of inter-departmental discussion and co-operation which is often required in order to deliver the best level of patient care. Shadowing a Consultant during his Cardiology outpatient clinics once a month since September has demonstrated the importance of asking specific questions and listening and observing well when the patient is responding in order to make an accurate diagnosis, and the need to make use of the most recent clinical studies.

My undergraduate degree in Biochemistry has provided me with a thorough knowledge of the life sciences which are fundamental to Medicine. Self-directed learning, particularly when working on my final project during my honours year, has enhanced my time management and organisational abilities and I have made use of my self-confidence and creative skills when delivering a number of presentations to my year group. An industrial placement year working for Delta Biotechnology, using the latest biotechnology research techniques to investigate sustainable ways to protect rice crops from fungal disease, involved working closely with others in my team, sharing information and finding ways to combine our individual skills effectively. My involvement in scientific research has also introduced

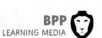

me to many of the ethical issues which occur in medicine, such as popular fears over genetic modification and the increasing power of big businesses within the pharmaceutical industry. During my Medicine degree I will be assisted by my experience of analysing complex data and statistics and I look forward to learning how to assimilate such research into an understanding of medical best practice. In particular I look forward to studying the role of genetics in neuro-psychiatric disorders and to learn how appropriate treatment can help those with life-limiting neurological disabilities. Becoming a doctor will allow me to serve the community through a vocation to which I truly aspire and I am committed to making full use of my time as a graduate student should I be offered this opportunity.

Postgraduate Personal Statement 3

The desire to become a doctor, combining both my humanitarian interests with my love of natural history, has been constant since childhood, and throughout my academic career I have been conscious of this ultimate goal. After suffering significant personal and family difficulties during my A level studies I did not achieve the three As required to meet my conditional offer to read Medicine, so I took the opportunity to study Physiology, an area of medical science which is of great interest to me. Although this was initially a setback, I have worked consistently hard throughout my degree in order to develop my academic skills and personal qualities to their full potential. This dedication helped me to gain funding for an MSc researching Neonatal Physiology which is now near to completion and my intention is to specialise in Clinical Neonatology in the future.

Studying Physiology has ensured I fully meet the requirements for graduate entry and, having achieved the university's prestigious Andrews Award for the highest results in my year group, as well as gaining a first class degree, I am confident that I have the scientific ability to continue this success on the MBBS programme. Critical thinking, analysis and problem-solving have been key elements to my success and I enjoy the challenge of integrating and interpreting disparate bodies of information in order to address research questions and meet clinical needs. Utilising my theoretical and research knowledge in a pressurised clinical environment, and communicating these complex ideas to patients and their families in a sensitive and accessible way, is one of the primary attractions of a career as a doctor; few careers offer this holy grail of combining challenge and responsibility with personal fulfillment and the chance to truly change people's lives, as well as opportunities for significant professional development.

Beyond my academic development, I believe my experience as a prospective mature student has allowed me to develop valuable interpersonal and management abilities. During my research degree I have been supervising a small team, ensuring everyone is kept up-to-date with progress and co-ordinating our day-to-day activities. I also have the strong communication skills required for daily interaction with the pharmaceutical and hospital staff involved in our project. Alongside my studies I have volunteered at hospital wards dedicated to the care of diabetic and stroke patients. As my role has been mainly to befriend patients and run errands to the shop and library for them, this has provided an important opportunity to work alongside nurses and allied health professionals and to develop my bedside manner. Conversations with everyone from first year medical students to Consultants has given me a fuller understanding of what a medical career entails and I have been moved by the dedication and commitment to patient care apparent at all levels within the hospital. Between my BSc and MSc I took a year out in order to work for a charity organising respite care for physically disabled children in some of the poorest areas of South Africa. This involved washing, feeding and dressing the children as well as accompanying them during daily events and helping them to access the activities at a level appropriate to them. Working with these children and their regular carers, who made so much of very limited financial resources, was a privilege and reinforced my commitment to working in a field where I can help others. Despite setbacks and the challenge of combining university study with voluntary work and a paid job, I have not deviated from my intention to become a doctor and I look forward to taking the next step towards achieving this.

Postgraduate Personal Statement 4

Having pursued a successful career as a Radiographer for several years, I now wish to develop the level of treatment I can offer my patients by training as a doctor. My employment experience enables me to make a realistic appraisal of the benefits, responsibilities and difficulties of a career in medicine, and I look forward to being in a position to bring together a breadth of knowledge in order to help others achieve their optimum health.

As a Therapy Radiographer I have had eight years' experience treating patients within NHS hospitals and

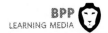

am therefore familiar with the typical hospital structure and organisation, and with the roles of the different members of a medical team. Working within Accident and Emergency and as part of the trauma team has ensured I fully understand the importance of clear communication, a calm but quick-witted approach and a commitment to being a co-operative and supportive team player. Computer technology has been an integral part of my daily workload and am I used to continually updating myself with the latest developments in image manipulation software. Teaching undergraduate medical students and Senior House Officers has given me a platform through which to share my enthusiasm for Radiology, as well as familiarising me with the content and standards of several sections of the MBBS programme. Part-time work in contract research for three years has given me an understanding of clinical drugs trials, including involvement in protocol development, reporting adverse events and conducting central laboratory diagnostic analysis. Participation at investigative meetings and frequent interaction with clinical staff has also given me a basic grounding in disease diagnosis and management.

My experience of managing a patient list will provide an authentic context to my studies, allowing me to link theoretical study with real life practice. I am confident that the professional skills I have developed, from training colleagues to managing my time effectively, will be an aid to my progress as a medical student. My first degree and subsequent experience has ensured I am familiar with the level of commitment required to succeed on a Medicine course and I am confident that I have the personal resilience and strong support network required to cope with the emotional, physical and academic demands of this training. During my degree I look forward to significantly widening my medical knowledge, as well as developing my diagnostic reasoning skills and ability to manage complex cases. In particular I look forward to utilising my real life knowledge of Radiography when studying Oncology and the diagnostic use of imaging. I will also relish the opportunity to discuss the theories behind recent developments in the NHS with my peers and, once qualified, I hope to be in a position to help shape the health service towards a more proactive and patient-orientated system at primary care level.

To relax I find landscape and natural history painting to be a useful creative outlet and, since a recent house move, have discovered a hidden passion for gardening and growing my own food. At university and throughout my career I have enjoyed involvement in several clubs and societies, at present acting as captain of a hospital football team and secretary of the Radiography Social Club. As an NHS professional with diagnostic and patient management experience, and a strong background in medical science, I am committed to making the most of this opportunity to further my professional development and I feel I have the qualities required to make a significant contribution to the medical world.

Postgraduate Personal Statement 5

Studying Medicine appeals to me as it combines a high level of patient interaction with the opportunity to utilise practical skills and theoretical research findings to address real life problems. During my undergraduate Chemistry degree I have enjoyed gaining the skills to work with a variety of tools and materials and to make logical, evidence-based deductions and I now wish to make use of these skills within the community as a doctor.

My first degree has provided a useful background to the Medicine modules on Pharmacology, Pathology and Biochemistry and completing this degree has involved assimilating large quantities of complex information, prioritising high workloads with strict deadlines and continually working at my full potential. My final year research project has given me confidence in the routine use of IT software such as model building programmes and advanced data banks and I have played a key role in conducting and presenting research as a team. Alongside report writing, this has enhanced both my oral and written communication skills and my ability to present ideas and results in an articulate and engaging way. Being awarded the university's year prize for Chemistry research has encouraged me in these endeavours and I intend to fully involve myself in clinical research as a doctor.

At university I have also developed the time management skills required to participate fully in the student community alongside my academic work. Captaining the hockey first team allows me to keep fit while developing my leadership and teamwork skills, supporting and encouraging the team regardless of the results of the match. In 2011, in my role as President of the One World Society, I took on the challenge of organising a Fair Trade Fair which was held over two weeks across the whole campus and which began an ongoing campaign for the university to gain Fair Trade status. This required me to co-ordinate several different teams, secure funding from local charities and businesses and publicise our efforts in local and national media. I have also held the positions of Social Secretary and Health and

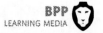

Safety Officer for the Student Union and I look forward to continuing similar activities at my next university as I feel they have helped me to become a more confident, poised and rounded person.

During two months of work experience at a GP's surgery I observed a range of procedures and consultations, giving me the chance to interact with hundreds of patients and to learn from the general practice team. Co-operative teamwork was much in evidence and the focus was very much on delivering the optimum care for patients at all times. Witnessing the doctors break bad news to patients and their families was an emotional experience and has prepared me for some of the harsher sides of medical practice. I also took the opportunity to learn from the doctors about the importance of having strong family or social support oneself and the benefits of releasing stress through hobbies and interests outside medicine. For the coming summer vacation I have arranged two weeks shadowing in several hospital departments in order to give myself a broader understanding of the NHS and of the almost limitless opportunities for specialist professional development available within medicine. I believe that I can offer my future university a mature, aware and self-motivated student, with a genuine commitment to the humanitarian aspects of medical practice. As a demanding and varied profession, medicine will offer me a wide choice of career paths with the opportunity for rapid development and I am confident I have the strength to take full advantage of these opportunities.

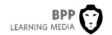

Postgraduate Personal Statement 6

While studying a degree in Clinical Sciences I have been fascinated to explore the social and biological aspects of health and the role of medical science in curing disease, relieving pain, saving lives and educating people to minimise the risk of illness and poor health. As a doctor I will have the opportunity to put such theoretical knowledge into practice and involve myself in improving others' wellbeing on a daily basis.

Throughout my degree I have nurtured a particular interest in human anatomy and I am also keen to enhance my understanding of human physiology in health and disease, as well as the social and behavioural aspects of Medicine. My previous degree and work experience will provide a context to my initial studies and I will employ the skills in IT, time management, teamwork and communication that I have built up as an undergraduate to ensure that I meet the challenges of the course. While conducting my dissertation research on bowel cancer in South America, for example, I overcame cultural and language barriers to convince the relevant men to undergo intensive interviewing and examination regarding a sensitive and stigmatised subject. This required tact, sensitivity and empathy, gaining the patients' trust and ensuring they understood the goals of the project and their own role. As an undergraduate I have enjoyed supplementing coursework with regular reading of medical journals and have learnt a great deal from these about medical law and ethics, topics I hope to explore further during the MBBS.

My four years' part-time employment as a care assistant at a residential home for people with Alzheimer's disease and dementia has confirmed my suitability for and

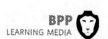

commitment to a career in medicine. While caring for, befriending and assisting the patients, I have developed confident and empathetic communication skills with both them and their families, gaining an understanding of the care requirements of those with high levels of dependency. My current voluntary role at a national asthma awareness organisation involves attending hospitals and clinics, talking to healthcare professionals and helping people to access the information they need. These roles, and my position as a nominated first aider at my Students' Union, have also involved extensive training, demonstrating my commitment to my own professional development. Recently I have taken up a position as a volunteer leader with the Cadets and this has helped me to learn about leadership and management, as well as allowing me to contribute to the community by encouraging young people to be active, motivated and self-disciplined.

Membership of the university's sailing club, five-a-side football team, and choral society has allowed me to build on my teamwork skills and has provided an active and creative balance to my academic studies. I have thoroughly enjoyed life on campus and I look forward to continuing to involve myself in the extra-curricular life of the university. As a mature student I have the experience to make a well-informed choice about my future and I feel the maturity and independence I have gained over the last three years will be of great assistance in allowing me to work to my full potential during my degree. My care experience has confirmed my enthusiasm and suitability for this career. I am fully committed to my ambition of becoming a Consultant specialising in Neurology, and I feel I have the skills and motivation to achieve this goal.

International Applicant Personal Statements

International Undergraduate Personal Statement 1

Medicine is a profession which, to me, is synonymous with challenge, dedication and the opportunity to positively impact people's lives. For as long as I can remember I have wanted to study Medicine because I thrive on situations which challenge me intellectually, emotionally and physically. About four years ago, due to the humanitarian emergencies in my continent, Africa, I became aware of 'Médecins Sans Frontières', and was struck by the commitment of the volunteer doctors. I have since followed their work in Nigeria, where they have Malaria and HIV/AIDS programmes. This has further increased my interest in human anatomy and the complex chemical interactions of the human body. I therefore hope to further my knowledge as soon as possible by going to medical school.

My choice of A level subjects has been geared towards the medical field. Chemistry has helped me improve on my analytical skills and the work it involves has made me more dedicated and focused. I find Physics challenging and chose Mathematics because I enjoy solving problems and logical thinking. Although the workload is high, I have been able to utilise various organisational skills taught by my teachers to properly structure my coursework. The time I spent volunteering in my school Community Development Programme provided me with the opportunity to serve in my local government Health Centre and the local government Home for Motherless Babies. This gave me the opportunity to work first-hand with ill and vulnerable people, helping

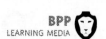

feed them, change their sheets and keeping them company. Volunteering at these institutions has also given me the chance to work closely with doctors and caregivers and to observe them in their work. It has also increased my communication skills and helped me to develop a sensitive attitude towards the needs of others.

Being appointed a School Prefect reinforced my sense of responsibility and positive attitude towards new things. The experience gave me the chance to be responsible for people younger than myself and in the process develop patience, rational thinking and teamwork; attributes I know are essential in medicine. Participation in various extra-curricular activities has also helped me become a more social person. As a member of the JETS (Junior Engineers, Technologists and Scientists) Club at my school, I took part in inter-school science-oriented competitions in which I won various prizes. I was the school chess champion for three consecutive years, gaining in the process the necessary discipline and analytical thinking essential for the study of Medicine. My hobbies include reading, art, crafts and photography, which have enabled me to develop skills in multi-tasking. My favourite books are autobiographies that tell of human triumphs over trials and I particularly find the books by Dr Benjamin Carson, an American Paediatric Neurosurgeon, inspirational. The difficulties he overcame in order to become a successful doctor give me faith that I can cope with the challenging, but rewarding, career that medicine provides.

Coming from four generations of university graduates makes me appreciate the benefits of a higher level education. This is a personal belief in a precious and unique heritage handed down to me. I look forward to making medicine my life's work and going to university will help me achieve this. University life sounds like a rewarding experience and I plan to get involved with photographic activities and settling in as a committed medical student.

International Mature Personal Statement 1

My motivation to study Medicine stems from a childhood incident in which doctors saved my uncle's life after he had a major heart attack. Observing the compassion and skill with which he was treated, and assisting in his care myself, inspired me to train to become a doctor and offer a similar level of care to others.

Science, especially Chemistry and Biology, interested me greatly at school and I am particularly interested in the way the sciences, Mathematics, IT and practical and social skills all come together in the practising of medicine. After spending two years following my school graduation earning money, I was inspired to get my career on track after hearing of my cousin in Sri Lanka passing his A levels and studying Medicine, despite the poverty of his community. To this end I have relocated to London and begun an 'Access to Medicine' course. Learning the basics of the relevant sciences has confirmed my ambition to utilise such knowledge in the diagnosis and treatment of medical conditions. I am making the most of this opportunity to prepare myself for a demanding degree course by developing my study skills.

My four weeks of work experience in a surgery in Germany gave me the opportunity to discuss career and training options with the healthcare professionals there. Through

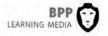

shadowing the doctor during consultations and operations I was able to learn some of the practical skills required and gain an insight into the social sacrifices associated with this career. I enjoyed interacting with the patients, learning about some of their conditions and treatments, and I observed the necessity for good communication between patients and their families, as well as within the medical team. Through shadowing doctors in the UK I have also been able to learn about the structure and function of the NHS.

Working in retail in a busy department store in Germany required me to develop excellent interpersonal skills to work effectively in a team to deliver high quality customer service to people of all ages and backgrounds. Similarly, my job in an insurance company has involved meeting and working with new people every day. A high standard of oral and written communication was needed as my duties included explaining the terms of insurance policies to people of all levels of understanding, as well as liaising with colleagues at different levels within the company. Often this was a highly pressurised environment with the need to show flexibility in switching frequently from one client appointment to another. Full-time employment has also demanded a high level of time management, organisation and IT skills, all of which should benefit me greatly at university.

In my free time I enjoy sports, football in particular, and during my captaincy, my football team has won several tournaments. Driving racing cars is another interest of mine and as the driver I have often had the ultimate responsibility for my team winning or losing. Both these positions have developed my ability to lead and motivate my peers, as well as providing a clear illustration of the value of teamwork. At school I also enjoyed writing and delivering speeches

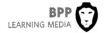

on stage, giving me confidence in performing in front of a large audience. To keep up with current issues in science I also watch scientific and medical documentaries.

Advice from my friends, and my own work experience, has allowed me to apply for Medicine with a realistic appreciation of both its demands and its rewards. I am fully committed to my ambition of working as a surgeon within the NHS and I feel I have the qualities and motivation to make the most of my time at university and achieve my goal.

International Mature Personal Statement 2

Medicine appeals to me as a way to use both science and compassion to help people through treatment, advice and reassurance. In my job as a healthcare assistant I have found there is a limit to the help I can give whereas in qualifying as a doctor I will have the knowledge and skills to provide a much higher level of care.

Having previously begun an Accountancy degree at university in Brazil I have experience of tertiary level study. Despite pressure from my family I found this was not the right career for me, but I enjoyed the opportunities to explore topics at a much higher level, to carry out independent research and learn from others in presentation groups. After this I left Brazil for the UK and began working towards my goal of becoming a doctor. Supplementing my school studies, I look forward to learning about the functions of the body, the basis for all further medical study. In particular I am interested in palliative care as it relates to Oncology as I feel the doctor's role in supporting cancer patients and

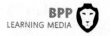

their family through potential bereavement is extremely important. The issues of Psychiatry and ethics are also fascinating to me, empathising with people with mental health problems and respecting patients' beliefs.

As a healthcare assistant I have enjoyed high levels of patient interaction and have been able to develop strong relationships with some individuals, learning about their diagnoses and treatments. Working in a team alongside a range of healthcare professionals, I have learnt about the demands and rewards of being a doctor. More than anything I have seen the importance of keeping patients informed about their treatment and condition, dealing compassionately with relatives, and communicating effectively with others on the medical team. My work has given me practical skills in manual handling, personal care, and measuring and recording details such as pulse rate and temperature. I now wish to increase my knowledge to a much higher level by studying Medicine. In a previous job as an administration assistant at a psychiatric hospital I typed transcripts of patient consultations. This allowed me to learn something of the range and characteristics of mental health problems, as well as highlighting the need for confidentiality.

My sense of fulfillment in helping people has led me to take part in support groups for people with weight problems. I was once overweight myself and I have been pleased to be able to support and encourage others by discussing my own experiences. This has improved my confidence as I became familiar with communicating with new people of all ages and backgrounds. I feel that my upbringing in total poverty in Brazil has been formative in my personal development as at the age of nine I began to help my mother with the housework and to work in my parents' shop. As a result

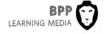

I am a responsible and determined person who is willing to work extremely hard. As a student and as an employee I am used to performing coolly under pressure; however, I also recognise my own limitations and am not afraid to ask for assistance when necessary. In times of stress I use my hobby of regular swimming to unwind and I also enjoy reading about different world cultures.

In the long term I hope to become a surgeon specialising in colorectal procedures. I am a well-motivated and hard working person and am fully committed to becoming a doctor. I intend to make the most of every opportunity available at university and I feel that I have the skills and dedication to make a positive contribution to society through medicine.

International Mature Personal Statement 3

My commitment to following a career in healthcare began during my childhood in Kenya, but despite high grades at school financial pressures meant my family could not afford for me to attend university. Instead, I trained as a nurse and have enjoyed a successful career within this profession, continually developing my skills through professional training. However, while my nursing career has brought me great satisfaction I have felt restricted by the limits on the level of specialist medical care I can provide. Having recently moved to the UK I have researched my career options thoroughly and I feel that the time is now right for me to make the most of the educational opportunities available here and pursue my original dream of training as a doctor.

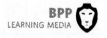

Success in my specialist field of Paediatric nursing has given me valuable experience of healthcare delivery and throughout my career I have taken pride in exploring the scientific knowledge and research underpinning my work. As a children's nurse I have close contact with families and carers and I am particularly enthusiastic about taking a holistic yet patient-centred approach to patient management, involving and supporting parents as necessary. My involvement in this area of work has provided enormous fulfillment and I feel it is also fundamental to the prognosis of the young patient. On a day-to-day basis I communicate with hundreds of people, from doctors, physiotherapists and social workers to cleaners, receptionists and janitors. Co-ordinating activities on my ward requires great organisation and effective communication between all members of staff. Although I am happy contributing to a dynamic and multi-disciplinary team, I am also experienced in taking the initiative and assessing problems on the ward as and when they arise. As well as dealing with all patients and families, including those undergoing very difficult circumstances, in a professional and tactful way, I also utilise my skills to manage resources in a logical and appropriate way. My recent experience as an agency nurse has introduced me to the NHS and given me a realistic understanding of the day-to-day challenges I will face.

As a specialist Paediatric nurse I have undertaken further training and acquired a sound understanding of areas of such as anatomy, physiology and pathology, particularly as they relate to children's developing bodies. This pursuit of specialist training has whetted my appetite for studying Medicine itself and has given me confidence in my ability to study at degree level. It has also ensured I am experienced in directing my own learning and helped to prepare me for future study. Given my background I am particularly looking forward to studying Paediatric Medicine and I am keen to further acquaint myself with the differences between theories of best practice in this field in the UK and Kenya. Reading journals such as the BMJ and BMC Medical Ethics keeps me informed about current developments within the field and I also enjoy wider scientific magazines such as New Scientist and Nature as these often present a different perspective on current themes within medical science. In my leisure time I enjoy keeping fit through attending the gym and running with a local club, and I find this helps to balance the pressures of working on a busy ward.

To conclude, in view of my related experience and deep commitment to practising as a doctor, I feel well prepared for the rigours of studying Medicine and the challenge of becoming a skilled and knowledgeable doctor.

International Postgraduate Personal Statement 1

As a mature student, my determination to study Medicine has taken me from Afghanistan, where my medical studies were interrupted, to my current 'Access to Medicine' course. My strong enthusiasm and interest in Medicine stems from a family background and also an aptitude for Biology, Chemistry and Mathematics. Medicine appeals to my deep appreciation for human life, together with studying man both as a human being and also as a biological machine. The decision to practise stems from a perpetual fascination with science combined with this basic love for life. When I began

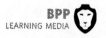

my undergraduate career, I had the opportunity to be exposed to the full range of medical courses, all of which reinforced and solidified my intense interest in studying Medicine. Having completed four years at Kabul Medical Institute and through my various work and voluntary experiences in the UK, I believe that I am in a unique position to study and practise Medicine. My ultimate goal is to obtain MRCS and FRCS training in Neurosurgery and I am also keen on doing research in the fields of Neurology.

At Kabul Medical Institute, I completed four years of study where I was considered an outstanding student. Working as a Doctor Assistant in Accident and Emergency, and in General Medicine and General Surgery, my clinical duties included sharing clerking of new medical admissions, observing and assisting senior doctors at out-patient clinic sessions and managing patients in CCU. I also attended ward rounds with senior doctors, performed procedures such as IV cannulation, nasogastic intubations and completed discharge summaries. In addition, I acted as a Health Advisor for the Swedish Committee for Logar, Afghanistan. This enabled me to realise that the practice of medicine entails more than remembering and dispensing scientific facts; that it requires exercising both mind and heart, along with genuine respect for life.

Working as a volunteer Health Advisor in the UK has given me an insight into the busy workings of a NHS Hospital and I have seen first-hand the importance of teamwork in providing healthcare. I have used my expertise in languages to work as an interpreter since 2008 for Health, Immigration, Legal and Social Services and since 2007 have worked as a carer for the disabled. This has enhanced my leadership, listening and communication skills and brought about the realisation that effective communication underpins effective patient care. I have a particular gift for empathising with people which was honed during my time in war torn Afghanistan where I dealt with people on a daily basis who had lost loved ones. During that time I learned a great deal about the reality of the medical profession.

In my spare time, I enjoy playing football and participated in all competitions at my previous medical school. I hope to carry on my interest in sporting activities at medical school as an outlet for the inevitable stresses of study. For relaxation, I enjoy listening to a variety of music and going to the cinema with my friends. Reading scientific magazines and journals has expanded my knowledge of current medical issues and given me a wider knowledge of some of the ethical issues in medicine today. Over time I have also undertaken computer courses as information technology is integral to patient care.

My range of experiences and personal aptitude has provided me with the perfect background with which to begin my studies; from the inspirational lessons of community service to the academic vigour of engaging in lab work. I look forward to the rewards of a career in medicine and transforming my success into direct aid for others by diagnosing and treating medical conditions and helping to maintain the health of my patients.

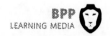

International Postgraduate Personal Statement 2

I have always had a great desire to help people and from a very early age the only career I have ever imagined is to be a hospital doctor. I have had the opportunity to study in the UK since moving here with my family in 2006, and would love the chance to pursue my studies further and fulfill my dream of becoming a doctor. My father is disabled and has a serious heart problem which has meant that I have been very involved in caring for him, accompanying him on hospital visits and providing practical and emotional support to my family. As my parents do not speak fluent English, from an early age I have acted as an interpreter between my father and the hospital doctors so that over the years I have learned excellent listening and communicating skills. Having been so involved with the hospital visits I have gained a lot of knowledge about how the doctors and other healthcare workers function as a team to provide the best care and treatment for patients.

My passion for science and medicine led me to study Molecular Medicine and it is my hope that the skills and knowledge I gained from my degree will provide an excellent basis on which to progress to a medical degree. There were many areas of this course that fascinated me, but I found the molecular signalling responses in the cardiovascular system particularly interesting and am very keen to study the heart and cardiovascular system further from a clinical prospective. To learn more about this area of medicine I am currently a volunteer at a busy Heart Failure Clinic where I gain a lot of satisfaction from talking to the elderly patients and helping out in any way I can. Through being involved with cardiac patients and my father's illness, I have observed, first-hand, how debilitating and wide-spread heart disease is. I would love to have the opportunity to study the anatomy, physiology and pathology of the heart as a medical student and hope to specialise in this area when I qualify as a doctor.

Since the age of 14 I have worked, part-time, as a waitress in a busy restaurant. This experience has helped me to develop my communication skills, as well as showing I can work well as part of a team, keeping patient and calm under sometimes stressful conditions. I was able to utilise these skills while undertaking voluntary work experience in the busy wards of Queen's Medical Centre University Hospital in 2011. I have learnt from talking to medical professionals, both in the UK and in my home country, Albania, that communication and teamwork are essential qualities of a good doctor, in addition to academic ability and compassion. My ability to remain focused under difficult circumstances is reflected by my excellent GCSE and A level results, as at this time I was supporting my father through an episode of serious ill health. I am very happy to have achieved a high level of fluency in four different languages as I know this will be an asset in my medical career. It is one of my ambitions to work overseas as a volunteer with 'Médecins Sans Frontières' in countries that are stricken by poverty and disease.

Although I am a hard-working, conscientious student, in my free time I enjoy socialising, going dancing and playing the piano. Playing basketball and volleyball keep me fit and I would hope to continue to these activities at university, as I know how important it is to maintain a balance between academic studies and recreational pursuits. I am fully aware of the high demands of the medical course but my passion for and commitment to medicine has only been strengthened by my experiences, and I am determined to realise my dream of one day becoming a doctor.

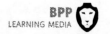

Chapter 8

Proofreading your Personal Statement

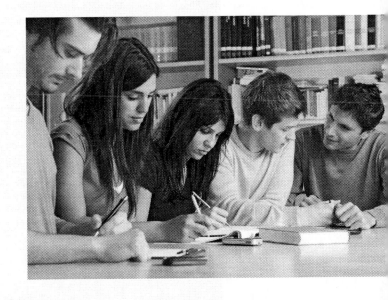

Proofreading your Personal Statement

When you believe that you are ready to submit your Personal Statement, **don't** until you are sure you are happy with its final format. It is also very useful to ask other people to read through your final version; it is amazing how helpful it is to obtain the viewpoint from 'a fresh pair of eyes'. For example, it may be very useful to receive the comments from an English teacher, especially with regard to your punctuation and writing style. Equally, there may be people you met during your work experience who would be pleased to help you in this way **but**, remember that at the end of the day it is **your** Personal Statement and if you feel passionate about an issue to the point that you are determined to include it, then do so!

Final checklist:

- Do you have a punchy and attention grabbing introduction?

- Do you come over as passionate about studying Medicine?

- Do you indicate that you have given serious practical consideration to the implications of establishing a medical career for you?

- Do you describe how your academic and extra-curricular activities have helped you to make this choice?

- Is every piece of information you provide clearly relevant to your application to study Medicine?

- Is your Personal Statement arranged in paragraphs? Is it balanced? Does it flow?

- Does your Personal Statement contain a concluding paragraph?

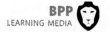

- Check all spelling and all punctuation.

Submitting your medical school application

The majority of medical school applications are submitted electronically. Your Personal Statement needs to be typed up electronically and must not exceed 47 lines and 4,000 characters (approx. 580 – 620 words, 12 Times New Roman).

If you are applying through your school or college, you will be provided with directions as to how to proceed. Those applying independently, such as graduates or mature students, can register directly on the UCAS website.

For more information visit **www.ucas.com**

KEY POINTS
- Keep looking for ways to **improve** upon your draft effort.

- Invite others to **proofread** your statement before you finally submit it.

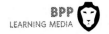

Chapter 9

Medical school Personal Statement: Things to avoid

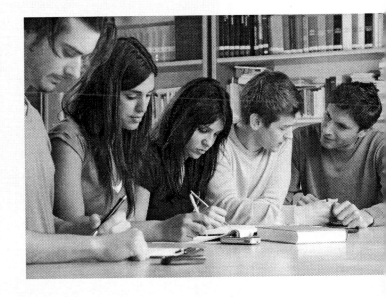

Medical school Personal Statement: Things to avoid

This guide has focused on helping you to draft, structure, refine and proofread your Personal Statement.

Here is a list of some things to avoid:

- Rushing the preparation of your Personal Statement – you will need plenty of time to write it!

- Needlessly repeating information that is contained in other parts of your application.

- Relying on a spell checking function – check it yourself; use a dictionary.

- Dishonesty, or deliberately misleading the reader.

- Using any word or phrase the meaning of which you are uncertain.

- Trying to be funny. Just play it straight.

- Drawing attention to any weakness, unless you have learnt from it, handled it, and become a more complete person.

- Including comments which criticise others or casting yourself in a favourable light in comparison to others.

- Simply listing achievements or interests; every comment must be relevant. Lists make for dry reading!

- Disjointed statements. Readers do not like having to flick backwards and forwards when trying to understand your comments.

- Overuse of the 'I' word.

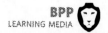

- Lack of structure; lack of paragraphs.

- Not proofreading your statement – ask your teachers, friends and family to help you in this regard. But remember that it is **your** Personal Statement!

KEY POINTS
- First, always make sure that your Personal Statement really is unique to you.

- Second, make sure you keep a copy. You can be sure that if you are called for interview, panel members are almost certain to question you specifically on some of the comments you have made. For you to say 'Oh, I forgot I wrote that' would give an incredibly bleak impression!

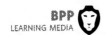

Chapter 10

Closing thoughts

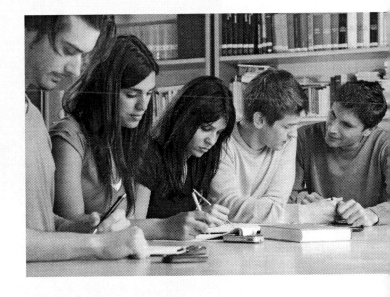

Closing thoughts

The aim of this guide is to provide you with a good idea of what should be included in your Personal Statement for application to medical schools in the UK. Our hope is that by following the principles and steps contained in this guide you will be able to compose a well-structured and effective Personal Statement.

We strongly recommend that you do seek more information from medical school websites and advice from staff at the medical school you wish to attend to ensure that your Personal Statement contains the information that they request.

From all of us at BPP Learning Media we would like to wish you every success in securing your place at medical school.

Good Luck!

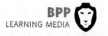

Appendix

Useful websites

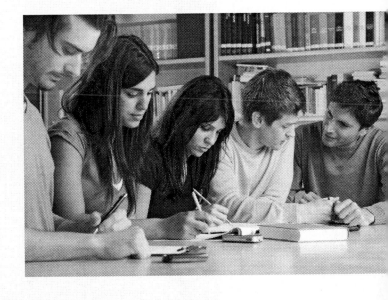

Useful websites

Universities and Colleges Admissions Service
www.ucas.com

Oxford Medical School
www.medsci.ox.ac.uk

General Medical Council
www.gmc-uk.org

Medical Schools Council
www.medschools.ac.uk

Entrance examinations
www.ukcat.ac.uk
www.bmat.org.uk
www.gamsat-ie.org

More titles in the Entry to Medical School Series

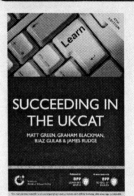

Nervous about the UKCAT? Want to know how you can improve your UKCAT score?

The UK Clinical Aptitude Test (UKCAT) is used by admissions staff as part of the application process to study Medicine or Dentistry at a UK University. With competition for places at an all time high it is crucial that you are fully prepared for this test. Advanced preparation is key to ensure that you know what to expect and achieve the best score possible.

This interactive guide, which contains practice questions and two complete mock tests, aims to help applicants, parents and teachers alike to prepare for and successfully complete the UKCAT. In this guide, the authors who have first hand experience of scoring highly in the UKCAT:

£14.99
March 2012
Paperback
978-1-445381-65-7

- Describe the context of the UKCAT within the application process

- Set out how to approach the five sections of the UKCAT: verbal reasoning, quantitative reasoning, ab-stract reasoning, decision analysis and non-cognitive test

- Provide practice questions for each section to work through as part of the learning process

- Explore time management techniques to ensure optimal performance

- In addition provide this guide contains two full mock exams to complete under test conditions

BPP
LEARNING MEDIA

Fully updated, this engaging, easy to use and comprehensive guide is essential reading for anyone serious about excelling in their UKCAT examination.

More titles in the Entry to Medical School Series

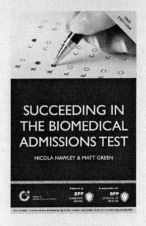

SUCCEEDING IN
THE BIOMEDICAL
ADMISSIONS TEST

NICOLA HAWLEY & MATT GREEN

£14.99

March 2012

Paperback

978-1-445381-64-0

The Biomedical Admissions Test (BMAT) is used by admissions staff as part of the application process for entry to a number of medical and veterinary schools in the UK. Places for these courses are heavily oversubscribed so it is vital that applicants excel in this test. Advanced preparation is key to ensuring that you know what to expect and to achieve the best score possible.

This interactive guide, which contains detailed guidance, practice questions and a complete mock test, aims to help applicants, parents and teachers alike to prepare for and successfully complete the BMAT. In this guide, Nicola Hawley and Matt Green:

- Describe the context of the BMAT within the application process

- Set out how to approach the three sections of the BMAT – namely the Aptitude and Skills, Scientific Knowledge and Applications and the Written task

- Provide practice questions for each section to work through as part of the learning process

- Explore time management techniques to ensure optimal performance

- In addition provide a full mock exam for readers to complete under test conditions

This engaging, easy to use and comprehensive guide is essential reading for anyone serious about excelling in their BMAT examination and successfully securing their place at university.

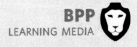

BPP
LEARNING MEDIA

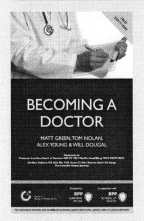
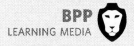

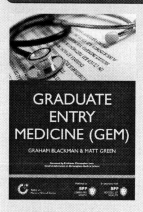
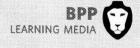

More titles in the Entry to Medical School Series

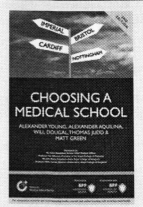

Choosing which Medical Schools to apply to is a decision that should not be taken lightly. It is important that you do your homework and consider carefully the many factors that differ between each institution.

This comprehensive and insightful guide written by medical students, for medical students, covers everything you need to know to enable you to select the Medical Schools best suited to you. The book is designed to help school leavers, graduates and mature individuals applying to Medical School, together with parents and teachers.

The first part of the book covers what to expect from life at medical school and things to consider prior to applying.

The second part then features chapters covering each individual UK Medical School. Each chapter is written by current medical students at the institution and is broken down into sections on the medical school, the university and the city finishing with the views of pre-clinical and clinical students.

This book is best used in conjunction with 'Becoming a Doctor'.

Key Features:

- **Forewords** - by Sir Liam Donaldson (Chief Medical Officer of England), Professor Ian Gilmore (President of Royal College of Physicians), Mr John Black (President of Royal College of Surgeons) and Professor Mike Larvin (Director of Education Royal College of Surgeons)

- **Insider Information** - An overview of what to expect from life at Medical School and tips for getting in and staying ahead

- **Latest Admission Statistics and Advice** - Up-to-date information on course structure, teaching methods, entrance requirements and other key factors to consider when choosing a Medical School

- **Pre-Medical and Postgraduate Advice** – views from preclinical and postgraduate students on getting in and what to consider

- **Easy Comparisons** - Quick comparison table covering each UK Medical School

- **Medical Education** - Clear sections focussing on pre-clinical and clinical education including summaries of teaching methods, support, examinations and teaching hospitals

- **Extracurricular Activities** - Information on what extracurricular opportunities are available at each Medical School and in the surrounding city

- **Students' Views** - Opinions and insights for each Medical School by current medical students

By using this engaging, easy to use and comprehensive guide, you will remove so much of the uncertainty surrounding how to best select the Medical Schools that are right for you.

£19.99
December 2011
Paperback
978-1-445381-50-3

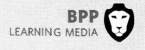

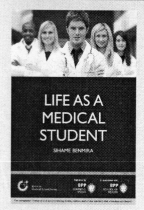
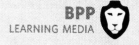